T0212664

SpringerBriefs in Public Health

SpringerBriefs in Public Health present concise summaries of cutting-edge research and practical applications from across the entire field of public health, with contributions from medicine, bioethics, health economics, public policy, biostatistics, and sociology.

The focus of the series is to highlight current topics in public health of interest to a global audience, including health care policy; social determinants of health; health issues in developing countries; new research methods; chronic and infectious disease epidemics; and innovative health interventions.

Featuring compact volumes of 50 to 125 pages, the series covers a range of content from professional to academic. Possible volumes in the series may consist of timely reports of state-of-the art analytical techniques, reports from the field, snapshots of hot and/or emerging topics, elaborated theses, literature reviews, and in-depth case studies. Both solicited and unsolicited manuscripts are considered for publication in this series.

Briefs are published as part of Springer's eBook collection, with millions of users worldwide. In addition, Briefs are available for individual print and electronic purchase.

Briefs are characterized by fast, global electronic dissemination, standard publishing contracts, easy-to-use manuscript preparation and formatting guidelines, and expedited production schedules. We aim for publication 8-12 weeks after acceptance.

More information about this series at http://www.springer.com/series/10138

Gary Jones

HIV and Young People

Risk and Resilience in the Urban Slum

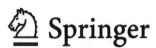 Springer

Gary Jones
James Cook University
Cairns
Queensland
Australia

ISSN 2192-3698   ISSN 2192-3701   (electronic)
SpringerBriefs in Public Health
ISBN 978-3-319-26813-2   ISBN 978-3-319-26814-9   (eBook)
DOI 10.1007/978-3-319-26814-9

Library of Congress Control Number: 2015958247

Springer Cham Heidelberg New York Dordrecht London

Printed on acid-free paper

Springer International Publishing AG Switzerland is part of Springer Science+Business Media
(www.springer.com)

Preface

This paper reviews the major findings regarding HIV and vulnerability. The fact is while global trends in HIV infection have diminished, some 30 years on into the epidemic, and a plethora of research that has guided policy and action, HIV remains a major threat to health and livelihood. The evidence amply demonstrates the multidimensional nature of HIV and the never static face of risk and resilience to infection and treatment uptake and the consistent vulnerability of certain groups often marginalised and disempowered. Gaps in the evidence emerge as fresh insights, and conceptual understandings develop and open up new areas of enquiry, along with global and contextualised changes in demographics and epidemiology, at the forefront of which is urbanisation and the informal slum settlement.

Sub-Saharan Africa carries the heaviest burden of HIV and takes its heaviest toll among young populations, as it has since the outset. Reflecting global trends, the continent is becoming younger. As cities in sub-Saharan Africa, and across the world, become increasingly youthful, young people are disproportionately impacted by HIV and routinely perform poorly across a wide spectrum of health indicators. As such, an association has been made between exponential urban growth and HIV infection. Young people hold the key in understanding where we are and where we expect to be in controlling global and urban epidemics, yet the least gains are being made in regard to young people, especially, concerning their sexual and reproductive health.

Much of the vulnerability of young slum dwellers, it is argued, owes to the subjective experience of humiliation felt at a deep level that impacts risky behaviour within the broader structural universe of informal settlement residence – poor shelter, violence, material deprivation, suboptimal health services and regular dislocation. Whereas the literature has comprehensively explained risky and health-enhancing behaviour largely through cognitive and social theory, the case is still being made in discerning young people's behaviour as a considered resilience, of purposeful behaviour aimed at dignifying life in the present and making good in a neglected and deprived environment. Such resilience may not be conceived or wish to be perceived as rational or productive. Life for young slum inhabitants by necessity is shown to be experimental in nature and has at its core immediate and diverse forms of gratification.

The connection between urban slum residence and perceptions of vulnerability, risk and resilience to HIV infection among young people residing and migrating to informal settlements is the broad area of interest for this review. This review examines HIV infection in a rapidly urbanising world and draws extensively on examples taken from Nairobi, Kenya and sub-Saharan Africa. Kenya now sits at the crossroads and is poised to become one of the few countries in the world to control its HIV epidemic. A focus on the national capital, Nairobi, provides an excellent example of how the future response to HIV will need to accommodate new forms of city space, deal with the rising number of young urban dwellers as well as the drastic intra-urban differences in slum and non-slum HIV prevalence and contextualise a response that can unravel the complexity of a mature, generalised and concentrated epidemic. For the purposes of in-depth analysis, it is also one of the few cities in sub-Saharan Africa that has provided insightful slum surveillance data of relevance to urban centres across the continent.

The literature review is structured as follows: section one is an introduction to the critical issues; section two sets the scene by exploring the literature on the subject of health and wellbeing, sexual and reproductive health in a rapidly urbanising world, including the structural determinants of health in urban slum settings, and the major theories which have sought to explain it; section three focuses on HIV within urban contexts globally, in sub-Saharan Africa and particularly in urban Kenya; section four reviews the available literature on youth vulnerability to HIV in the urban slum and explores the key dynamic of gender and gender relations; section five presents the case for urban migration and the very special set of needs and vulnerability faced by the legions of young people taking up residence in the urban slum; and section six concludes by outlining the most pressing gaps in the evidence as demonstrated from the literature and identifies research priorities required to significantly address these shortcomings.

Cairns, QLD, Australia   Gary Jones

Keywords HIV • Urban slums • Vulnerability and risk • Resilience • Dignity and humiliation • Self-perception • Risky behaviour • Sub-Saharan Africa • Kenya

Acknowledgements

The author thanks the following: PhD Supervisory Team at the Cairns Institute, notably, Professors Komla Tsey and Deborah Graham for overall guidance and direction in the production of this work; helpful input from Alexis Martin (Writing Consultant) and Jani de Kock (First Person, South Africa), respectively, for the literature review narrative and research methodology; Dr. Blessing Mberu (Africa Population and Health Research Center) for helping to conceptualise the need and purpose of this book; Dr. Evelin Lindner (World Dignity University) for clarity concerning the study of human dignity and humiliation; and colleagues at the Kenya UNAIDS Country Office and UNAIDS Regional Support Team for Eastern and Southern Africa for their ongoing encouragement.

About the Author

Gary Jones is a research scholar at the Cairns Institute, James Cook University, studying for a Doctorate in Philosophy (Society and Culture), 2014–2017.

Contents

Chapter 1
Introduction

Abstract This chapter provides a broad overview of the key issues regarding HIV and young people in the context of African urban slum life, in particular, conceptual understandings of vulnerability, risk and resilience and the interpersonal role of dignity and humiliation in shaping perception and behaviour.

Keywords HIV • Urban slums • Vulnerability and risk • Resilience • Dignity and humiliation • Self-perception • Risky behaviour • Sub-Saharan Africa • Kenya

Vulnerability, Risk and Resilience

Vulnerability is a complex construct. Complex because its conceptual understanding is never absolute and evolves overtime, between social groups and according to context. Vulnerability is a relative state, a multifaceted continuum between resilience and helplessness (World Bank 2015) and given meaning through subjective perception (Kahneman and Krueger 2006). For this paper, vulnerability is defined as the degree to which a person is susceptible to HIV infection. A person's vulnerability is determined by a combination of biomedical and behavioural factors, including physiology, gender, age, education and peer influence, and it is shaped by the totality of the external environment (Cluver et al. 2014).[1]

For this literature review, risk is defined as exposure to the HIV and probability of infection. Whereas vulnerability involves external structural factors largely beyond the control of the individual, 'taking risks' refers more to purposeful behaviour, of individual agency, and the likelihood of acquiring HIV through a given event or series of acts.[2] The risk of HIV infection is affected by factors of vulnerability and the consequences of a given act. The two positions are inextricably linked.

---

[1] Vulnerable has been defined as: '… open to attack, injury or criticism…' (*The Little Oxford Dictionary* 1998, p. 745).

[2] Risk has been defined as: '…chance of danger, injury, loss…' (*The Little Oxford Dictionary* 1998, p. 559).

© The Author 2016
G. Jones, *HIV and Young People: Risk and Resilience in the Urban Slum*,
SpringerBriefs in Public Health, DOI 10.1007/978-3-319-26814-9_1

1

In being vulnerable, there is always the probability of a negative (health) outcome. Vulnerability and risk are rooted in a significant lack of welfare that goes beyond socially accepted norms and is shaped by an episode or series of events in which the result is not certain (World Bank 2015). The magnitude, frequency, duration and scope of risk and stress, as experienced by individuals, households and communities, form the structural basis of vulnerability (Ludi and Bird 2007). Much of the research accepts that vulnerability is a multilayered phenomenon and best understood through two interlinked sides representing external and internal factors as made clear by Chambers (1995). The former side refers to exposure to shocks, stress and risk and the latter, a basic defencelessness and incapacity to act without incurring damage or loss (Chambers 1995).

Throughout the literature, the concept of vulnerability is entwined with notions of risk and resilience, which is oftentimes not made explicit. Furthermore, resilience is often associated with notions of dignity, in particular, how certain behaviour serves to dignify life and wellbeing for an individual or community. What the literature does not make clear is the many and often conflicting perceptions of dignity and health, born in part from a multitude of interpretation of what is vulnerability and what is risk, and, furthermore, what actually constitutes 'health'. Being vulnerable, for most of the literature, implies a state of dependency, which may not be reliable or consistent, and therefore inherently 'undignifying'. Dignity and resilience are often seen as highly emotive terms and can blur the rigours of academic enquiry. In this review, in depicting the social universe for young slum dwellers, where necessary, a distinction is made between the numerous constructs relevant to a discussion of vulnerability, risk and resilience.

The literature has highlighted the need to distinguish between self-perceived risk and self-perceived vulnerability (Bradley et al. 2011). Self-perception of risk is best understood as the likelihood of becoming HIV infected based on knowledge and behaviour, and self-perceived vulnerability concerns felt susceptibility to HIV even in the absence of risk behaviour (Bradley et al. 2011). Though interwoven, the constructs of risk and vulnerability and the role of self-assessment are key to understanding subjective interpretation and behaviour patterns regarding the transmission of HIV (Bradley et al. 2011). Far less explored is the self-assessment of dignity and humiliation by vulnerable young slum-dwelling populations in the context of risk, resilience and HIV.

HIV, Risk and Resilience

No one is immune to HIV (Power 2013). Everyone is vulnerable to contracting HIV; the question is to what extent. For people accessing and using the full gamut of prevention, treatment, care and the extensive range of support services, the likelihood of acquiring HIV is perceived, for the better part, as an 'acceptable risk' (Hunter and Fewtrell 2001). The literature demonstrates that for many slum-dwelling inhabitants of sub-Saharan Africa, where HIV and AIDS have from the outset exacted its greatest toll, vulnerability and risk compound and that knowledge, perception and purposeful action against acquiring HIV remain limited.[3]

Individual and collective resilience, here, is the ability to safeguard against (re-) infection or recover from the outcome of risky behaviour, of being HIV positive and of navigating the uncertainty of social change in the face of hardship, set back and threat to life and livelihood.[4] As Lever states (2010), effective personal resilience is sustainable over time and enables individuals to draw on vital resources including external means of support. In response to threat, perceived or actual, the evidence demonstrates that negative coping mechanisms are often deployed by different groups at different times and in different circumstances which, while dealing with the immediate problem, put at risk long-term health and wellbeing (Degenova et al. 2010). This choice of action can also be understood as an attempt to salvage a sense of dignity in the face of uncertainty, want and resignation.

Constructing conceptual understanding of vulnerability, risk and resilience is an integral part of modelling health and wellbeing at all levels of service delivery. Underpinned by theoretical persuasion, modelling formal and informal health care reflects an understanding of the nature of and motive for patterns of human behaviour (United States Department of Health and Human Services 2002). In some cases, either wittingly or unwittingly, these models draw on principles from different perspectives of social theory. Arguably, this is not surprising as efforts continue to craft an 'ideal type' of risk and behaviour and to more comprehensively profile modern urban vulnerability.[5] The efficacy of mainstream approaches of both health education and health promotion has been questioned in the face of a continuing HIV epidemic which can, in essence, be controlled if not eradicated (Joint United Nations Programme on HIV/AIDS (UNAIDS) 2014b).

Broadly, two principal health models, social learning theory and the structural-environmental paradigm, have formed key theoretical perspectives in explaining reproductive and sexual behaviour (King 1999). In practical terms, these positions are not mutually exclusive (United States Department of Health and Human Services 2002). Sexuality and risky behaviours, as best described by structural-environmental

---

[3] 'HIV stands for 'human immunodeficiency virus'. HIV is a virus (of the type called retrovirus) that infects cells of the human immune system (mainly CD4 positive T cells and macrophages—key components of the cellular immune system), and destroys or impairs their function. Infection with this virus results in the progressive deterioration of the immune system, leading to 'immune deficiency'. The immune system is considered deficient when it can no longer fulfil its role of fighting off infections and diseases. Immunodeficient people are more susceptible to a wide range of infections, most of which are rare among people without immune deficiency. Infections associated with severe immunodeficiency are known as 'opportunistic infections', because they take advantage of a weakened immune system...AIDS stands for 'acquired immunodeficiency syndrome' and is a surveillance definition based on signs, symptoms, infections, and cancers associated with the deficiency of the immune system that stems from infection with HIV' (UNAIDS 2008, p. 1).

[4] Resilient has been defined as: '...recovering from setback' (*The Little Oxford Dictionary* 1998, p. 550).

[5] 'Ideal type, in the social sciences, refers to an artificially constructed 'pure type' which emphasizes certain traits of a social item which do not necessarily exist anywhere in reality' (McLeish 1993).

theory, are based in individual, social, structural and environmental factors that provide a framework, inter alia, for analysing the context of adolescent reproductive behaviour (McLeroy et al. 1988; Sweat and Denison 1995). Work on identifying core drivers of vulnerability has been informed by the study of dignity and humiliation (Hartling et al. 2013; Lindner 2012). This work notes the pervasive impact of humiliation and related self-conscious emotions, in particular, 'shame', experienced as an interpersonal and inter-relational event and its impact on risk-taking behaviour.[6] However, as proponents state, the empirical base is still lacking and requires further investigative work and especially so across diverse settings (Hartling 2005; Shultziner and Rabinovici 2011).

Research into dignity and humiliation needs to first unravel the complexity of urban life. The nexus of vulnerability, risk and resilience has been captured by the World Health Organization (WHO) and the United Nations Habitat agency (UN-Habitat) through the development of a framework for the study of urban habitation. The framework sees each aspect largely determined by a complex mix of physical, emotional, social and economic factors which can be understood from four classifications relevant to urban wellbeing: first, 'natural and built environment'; second, 'social and economic environment'; third, 'food security and quality'; and fourth, 'services and emergency health management' (WHO and UN-Habitat 2010, p. xi). The framework provides a classification for the study of dignity and humiliation in which the multiplicity of factors directly relating to health and wellbeing are understood by analysing the dynamic relationship and influence that each part holds over the other.

Young People, Urbanisation and HIV

For HIV and AIDS, understanding the link between young people's vulnerability and their sexual and reproductive health is paramount. Young people, of all age cohorts, are at the centre of the HIV epidemic with the primary mode of transmission, across Sub-Saharan Africa, being heterosexual sex (Mberu 2012).[7] Young people below the age of 25 now account for around 50 per cent of all new global HIV infections, and in many developing countries, notably sub-Saharan Africa, as much as 60 per cent of all new infections are among the 15–24 age group with females greatly outnumbering males and, in some contexts, by a factor of 2:1

---

[6] Humiliation has been defined as 'causing someone to feel ashamed and foolish by injuring their dignity and self-respect' (*Oxford Dictionaries*, Oxford University Press, 2015); and dignity has been defined as 'the state or quality of being worthy of honour or respect' (*Oxford Dictionaries*, Oxford University Press, 2015).

[7] For young people, age group conceptualizations are: 'childhood,' any person under the age of 18 (United Nation Human Rights Office of the High Commissioner for Human Rights (UNOHCHR) 1989), 'adolescence' referring to the age group 10–19 years (WHO) and 'youth' the 15–24 age group (political instruments of the United Nations); young people, less formally defined, include both adolescents and young adults, the 10–24 age group (Mberu 2012).

(Mberu 2012). Women below the age of 25 years are at most risk of contracting HIV; in sub-Saran Africa, adolescent girls are the most vulnerable to HIV and account for one in four new HIV infections (UNAIDS 2014a). For urban women, HIV is 1.5 times higher than for urban men and 1.8 times higher than rural women (WHO and UN-Habitat 2010). Whereas there is an overall global decline in AIDS-related deaths, UNAIDS reports that adolescents are the only age group in which AIDS-related deaths have not decreased (UNAIDS 2014a). This situation is striking not just for public health but also for the threat to inalienable human rights given that HIV-positive adolescents require lifelong treatment and must prepare to face the various forms of humiliation owing to the stigma of simply being HIV positive.

HIV continues to threaten lives of individuals and their livelihoods, the security of families, however defined, and wellbeing of entire communities (UNAIDS 2014b). In Africa, the leading cause of death for adolescents is AIDS related; globally, it is the second highest cause of death for the same age group (UNAIDS 2015). In Kenya, an estimated 17 per cent of all AIDS-related deaths are among adolescents and youth (Ministry of Health, Kenya 2012).[8] HIV discriminates against most vulnerable populations – vulnerable because of circumstance, personal traits, disposition, social networks and structural determinants (United States Agency for International Development (USAID) 2012). These vulnerable or 'key populations' are the focus of concerted global action to reduce global HIV incidence. The evidence shows that many key populations concentrate in urban environments (UNAIDS 2014c). Their vulnerability and resilience are not static but evolve according to context, time and place. Daily life, often described as 'survival' for many of these marginalised groups, is learned in situ as well as how to gain an advantage often against overwhelming odds.

Urban Slums as Settings for Risk and Vulnerability

Urban spaces are expanding and patterns of urban life constantly change. Seen as the engine for industrialisation, economic development and social advancement, urban centres are best seen as a 'blessing and a curse' given that within the urban context there are concentrations of poverty, slum growth and social disruption (United Nations Fund for Population (UNFPA) 2007). Vlahov et al. (2007) have described the urban slum as a 'concentration of disadvantage' in which population-level patterns of sickness and health are routinely formed by structural factors. As such, slum settlements reflect the urbanisation of poverty and constitute

---

[8] 'In epidemiology, prevalence refers to the proportion of a population having an identified condition, such as HIV/AIDS. Through comparing the total number of people with that condition and number of people in that population group the extent of prevalence can be determined; incidence is a measure of the risk of a condition developing in a specific period of time' (Sifiris and Myhre 2015).

ever-evolving urban 'risk spaces' (Fitzpatrick and LaGory 2000). Humiliation, it is argued, feeds off such situations of poverty and disconnection (Lindner 2009, 2012). There are, however, gaps in the empirical evidence on how this sense of poverty and entrapment is internalised and given expression especially in the African slum. Whereas consistent exclusion from social services is well noted as a factor leading to humiliation and shame (Lindner 2006), its effect on vulnerability in the urban context still needs to be developed through concerted empirical evidence. Moreover, much of the research into urban vulnerability is still dominated by an approach which adopts an economic analysis of poverty and in so doing fails to appreciate the complex reality of poor people which is by essence diverse, dynamic and multifaceted (Chambers 1995).

It is reckoned that approximately 54 per cent of the global population now lives in urban settings (United Nations 2014). With annual growth rate of urban dwellers at 3.4 per cent between 2005 and 2010, and 4.8 per cent in 2013, Africa is growing at a pace unrivalled elsewhere in the world (Aribisala 2013; Hove et al. 2013). In Sub-Saharan Africa, it is estimated that between 2000 and 2013, the urban population would double (UNFPA 2007). Within Africa, East Africa provides the most extreme case of population growth with one of the highest growth rates in the world (Aribisala 2013). In Kenya, the population is expected to grow from the current 43 million to more than 100 million by 2050 (Aribisala 2013). In sub-Saharan Africa, nearly half (45 per cent) of people living with HIV now reside in urban areas (UNAIDS 2014c). Based on global estimates of demographic trends and patterns of infection, ending AIDS, it is now widely held, will largely be won or lost in the cities.

The demographic profile of urban populations is changing and, in Africa, becoming increasingly younger. Africa is believed to have the youngest population in the world with an estimated 200 million Africans between the ages of 15–24. In Kenya, 43 per cent of its population is under 15 years (Aribisala 2013). This has been described as the Youth Bulge[9] (Sommers 2011). By 2030, it is estimated that approximately 60 per cent of all urban dwellers will be under the age of 18 (UN-Habitat 2014a). Population dynamics changes the shape and creates new forms of urban risk and vulnerability. Mberu (2012) note that research is being challenged to keep apace of these developments, and particularly so regarding attitude and behaviour among urban youth. The literature reveals that insight into the subjective interpretation of vulnerability and resilience remains wanting overall, and notably so for urban youth.

In understanding the drivers of HIV, 'place matters' (UNAIDS 2011b). The place of residence, work and social mixing, along with age and gender, provides the global framework for understanding and addressing vulnerability, including HIV infection (WHO and UN-Habitat 2010). Place is shown to be a major determinant of health and wellbeing in a myriad of ways. Areas with the poorest health out-

---

[9] In many sub-Saharan African countries, young people represent the majority share of the population pyramid. The term 'youth bulge' is often used in the context of 'social instability', given the lack of appropriate age-friendly social services and economic opportunities.

comes are those where the poorest people live and work (WHO and UN -Habitat 2010). Descriptive statistics on the epidemic only have meaning when sufficiently disaggregated, especially concerning gender, age and location. But, as the literature shows, this is very often not the case in national and subnational records on HIV and AIDS. Much of the demographic and ethnographic data on urban settings do not take into account profound differences between slum, intra-slum and non-slum set- tlement, a situation described as the 'curse of aggregates' (Lamba 1994). The litera- ture broadly holds that there will be little progress in improving health outcomes in urban settings without first providing detailed and disaggregated data inclusive of socioeconomic profile and geographical areas involving applied research targeting the different forms of urban slums.

As UN-Habitat states (2007), sub-Saharan Africa urban growth is driven by expansion of the different forms of slum settlement.[10] For many least developed countries, rapid urbanisation is largely owing to exogenous factors and not a natural, evolutionary movement towards modernity (Jorgenson and Rice 2012). As Arimah's research shows (2010), a large part of the urban poor is increasingly found in the various types and forms of slum settlements. In Africa, 55 per cent of all urban- residing populations now live in a slum (UN-Habitat 2014b). The fact that a higher than expected proportion of people inhabits urban areas relative to concurrent levels of economic development has been described as 'over-urbanisation' (Smith 1987). In terms of unearthing the reality of life in the slum, data collection still proves a global challenge not least as most of the available information on slum dwellers needs further disaggregation (UN-Habitat 2007).

Cotton (2013) explained how life in the slum is harsh with residents facing mul- tiple hazards to health shaped by factors of age, gender, ethnicity, race and/or disability and socio-economic status. Slum areas are typically characterised by exclusion, including lack of land rights and access to infrastructure, public facilities and basic services (UN-Habitat 2011). Unlike their urban counterparts, slum dwell- ers are largely excluded from the 'urban advantage'[11] and instead face persistent challenges of unemployment, pollution, traffic, crime, high cost of living and com- petition over scarce resources (UNICEF 2012). The literature, however, fails to adequately depict how these same residents seek to realise their personal sense of 'urban advantage' and in so doing dignify their life in the slum nor has research holistically and consistently enquired into possible links between dignity, resilience and social status. The innovation of slum-dwellers and the strength of their social capital is a significant but often neglected feature of urban studies (UN-Habitat 2006b). Empirical enquiry that explores the notion of seeking dignity through inno-

---

[10] For this review, unless otherwise specifically stated by a cited source, the words slum and infor- mal settlement are used to refer to all types of suboptimal living conditions.

[11] The concept of urban advantage holds that cities are the main setting for progress and that the urban space facilitates the advancement of political ideas and action and provides unlimited ben- efits for the best level of health, education and public services, like adequate supplies of water and sanitation.

vation and initiative notably for young people is weak and overwhelmingly missing in the research of African urban slum life.

Slum-dwellers, and especially those living in extreme poverty, have been variously described as 'populations of humanitarian concern' because for many securing the basic necessities to sustain life and livelihood is never certain. In the urban setting, populations of humanitarian concern are heterogeneous and include long-term multi-generation residents, economic migrants, internally displaced persons and refugees fleeing humanitarian crisis (International Office for Migration (IOM) 2011). Given the continuing exponential growth of cities, the United Nations International Strategy for Disaster Reduction (UNISDR 2014) points to the evolving urban dynamic as critical for global efforts in disaster risk reduction. Moreover, given current patterns of urbanisation and in particular the unplanned urban settlement, it is held that vulnerabilities to loss of life and livelihood and attrition of social, economic and environmental assets are expected to continue and likely increase (UNISDR 2014).[12] This assumption has immediate implications for discussions on sociopolitical power dynamics as well as the role of social capital in accessing life-saving resources, all of which are shown to be core components for managing vulnerability and reducing risk. The sprawling urban settlements of Nairobi are a case in point.

As the evidence demonstrates, in eastern and southern Africa, slum inhabitants face vast health inequities, as well as heightened vulnerability to a wide range of disease and illness, including HIV (WHO and UN-Habitat 2010). In the Nairobi slums, the average HIV prevalence for women aged 15–49 years living in a non-slum area is 8.4 per cent, while the same cohort living in the slum is 12.4 per cent; similarly for men of the same age group, prevalence in the non-slum is 2.9 per cent, and for men residing in the slums, it is 5.7 per cent (Africa Population and Health Research Centre 2014; Kenya National AIDS & STI Control Programme and Ministry of Health 2013; Madise et al. 2012). For all of Nairobi County, adult preva-

---

[12] For UNISDR (2012), the 'Ten Essentials for Making Cities Resilient' are '1. Put in place organisation and coordination to understand and reduce disaster risk, based on participation of citizen groups and civil society. Build local alliances. Ensure that all departments understand their role in disaster risk reduction and preparedness. 2. Assign a budget for disaster risk reduction and provide incentives for homeowners, low-income families, communities, businesses and the public sector to invest in reducing the risks they face. 3. Maintain up-to-date data on hazards and vulnerabilities, prepare risk assessments and use these as the basis for urban development plans and decisions. Ensure that this information and the plans for your city's resilience are readily available to the public and fully discussed with them. 4. Invest in and maintain critical infrastructure that reduces risk, such as flood drainage, adjusted where needed to cope with climate change. 5. Assess the safety of all schools and health facilities and upgrade these as necessary. 6. Apply and enforce realistic, risk-compliant building regulations and land use planning principles. Identify safe land for low-income citizens and upgrade informal settlements, wherever feasible. 7. Ensure that education programmes and training on disaster risk reduction are in place in schools and local communities. 8. Protect ecosystems and natural buffers to mitigate floods, storm surges and other hazards to which your city may be vulnerable. Adapt to climate change by building on good risk reduction practices. 9. Install early warning systems and emergency management capacities in your city and hold regular public preparedness drills. 10. After any disaster, ensure that the needs of the affected population are placed at the centre of reconstruction, with support for them and their community organisations to design and help implement responses, including rebuilding homes and livelihoods'.

lence is estimated at 8 per cent, compared with 6 per cent for the rest of the country (APHRC 2014; Madise et al 2012; Nairobi City Council 2014).

Approximately 34 per cent of Kenya's population now lives in urban areas, and more than 75 per cent reside in informal settlements that occupy some 5 per cent of the total land mass (APHRC 2014; Integrated Regional Information Networks 2013; UN-Habitat 2005). These slum areas have rarely figured in urban plans and largely go unrecognised, growing spontaneously on available land inside the city or on its outskirts (Pamoja Trust 2009). For Pamoja Trust (2009) it is a straightforward case of disenfranchisement and alienation of slum dwellers. Exclusion, experienced personally or collectively, for Lindner (2010), is very often a precursor of humiliation. Kenya's annual informal settlement growth rate is estimated at 5 per cent, making it one of the highest in the world and the number of urban slum dwellers is expected to double over the course of the coming 15 years (UN-Habitat 2005).

Nairobi, Kenya

Strongly influenced by factors of migrancy, trade and commerce, the HIV epidemic in Kenya, the fourth largest in the world, is closely linked with that of sub-Saharan Africa, which accounts for almost 70 per cent of the global total of new HIV infections annually (UNAIDS 2014a). Nairobi provides an excellent case study of African urban risk and development. With a population of around 3.36 million estimated in 2011, Nairobi, the second largest city by population in the African Great Lakes region, contributes to approximately 60 per cent of the country's GDP and is growing at 2.9 per cent per annum (Central Intelligence Agency 2015). Nairobi, the nation's capital, is a hub for business enterprise, for health innovation, and is described as a leading African city, both politically and financially (Bauck 2015). Nairobi is equally seen as a leading social centre in the region (Global and World Cities 2015).

While Nairobi is home to much wealth and economic activity, there is also conspicuous inequality and it has two of Africa's three largest slums – Kibera and Mathare (UNAIDS 2014c). With a notable lack of equity in Kenya, and particularly in Nairobi, it was earlier reckoned that one-third of Kenya's urban population was living below the national poverty line (UN-Habitat 2006a). In its global report (2006b), UN-Habitat stated that the Kenya Gini Coefficient is 0.45 and in Nairobi 0.59 and that inequality is more pronounced in Nairobi than elsewhere in the country, with an estimated 45 per cent of Nairobi's income going to 10 per cent of the city population and the poorest 10 per cent sharing in 1.6 per cent of the total city's income (UN-Habitat 2006a). A sense of resignation from living in extreme poverty can be a factor leading to humiliation owing in part to notions of powerlessness in not being able to alter individual or community circumstance which can lead, in turn, to episodes of physical and mental illness (Lindner 2010).

Kenya is home to tens of thousands of migrant and mobile populations including refugees and internally displaced people, housed in formal camp settings, or more informally across the country and often in urban centres, notably Nairobi. In Kenya, the total 'population of concern' stands at over half a million people (United Nations Office for the Coordination of Humanitarian Action (UN/OCHA) 2015).

Neighbouring countries include Somalia and South Sudan, categorised as 'very high-risk' states (Haken et al. 2014) and currently characterised by cyclical violence, social upheaval and mass displacement of people across international borders. It is thought that about two-thirds of the refugees and asylum seekers in Kenya have fled general insecurity in their respective countries of origin since the 1990s (UN/OCHA 2015). South Sudan is suspected of having an emerging HIV epidemic (Sudan Tribune 2014) which has immediate and long-lasting implications for the AIDS response in Kenya. Each person caught up in displacement and involuntary movement has an account of personal and institutional vulnerability and a sense of resilience having made it this far.

References

African Population and Health Research Center. (2014). Population and health dynamics in Nairobi's informal settlements. Report of the Nairobi Cross-sectional Slums Survey (NCSS) 2012. Nairobi: African Population and Health Research Center.

Aribisala, F. (2013, October 11). Population growth and control in Africa. *The Hub: International Perspectives.* Retrieved from https://www.stratfor.com/the-hub/population-growth-and-control-africa

Arimah, B. (2010, January). *The face of urban poverty explaining the prevalence of slums in developing countries* (Working Paper No. 2010/30). Retrieved from https://www.researchgate.net/publication/46474265

Bradley, H., Tsui, A., Hindin, M., Kidanu, A., & Gillespie, D. (2011). Developing scales to measure perceived HIV risk and vulnerability among Ethiopian women testing for HIV. *AIDS Care, 23*(8), 1043–1052. doi:10.1080/09540121.2010.543880.

Bauck.com (2015). City Guide to Nairobi - The Green City in the Sun. Retrieved from http://www.bauck.com/nairobi-city-guide-green-city-sun/

Central Intelligence Agency. (2015). *Major urban areas-population.* Retrieved from https://www.cia.gov/library/publications.the-world-factbook/fields/2219.html

Chambers, R. (1995). Poverty and livelihoods: whose reality counts? *Environment and Urbanization, 7*(1), 173–202. Retrieved from http://eau.sagepub.com/content/7/1/173.full.pdf

Cluver, L. D., Orkin, F. M., Boyes, M. E., & Sherr, L. (2014). Cash plus care: Social protection cumulatively mitigates HIV-risk behaviour among adolescents in South Africa. *AIDS, 28*(Suppl 3), 389–297. doi:10.1097/QAD.0000000000000340.

Cotton, C. (2013). *Research to practice – Strengthening contributions to evidence-based policy making.* Retrieved from https://www.mcqil.ca/isid/files/isid/pd2013otton.pdf

DeGenova, M. K., Patton, D. M., Jurich, J. A., & MacDermid, S. M. (2010). Ways of coping among HIV-infected individuals. *The Journal of Social Psychology, 134*(5), 655–663. Retrieved from http://www.tandfonline.com/doi/abs/10.1080/00224545.1994.9922996#.VeUnxXnos-U

Fitzpatrick, K., & LaGory, M. (2000). *Unhealthy places: The ecology of risk in the urban landscape.* New York: Routledge.

Globalization and World Cities Research Network. (2015). *Nairobi.* Retrieved from http://en.wikipedia.org/wiki/globalizationandWorldcitiesResearchNetwork

Haken, N., Messner, J. J., Hendry, K., Taft, P., Lawrence, K., Brisard, L., & Umaña, F. (2014). *Fragile states index, 2014. The fund for peace publication.* Retrieved from CFSIR1423: www.fragilestatesindex.org

Hartling, L. (2005). *Humiliation: Real pain, a pathway to violence.* Retrieved from http://www.cchla.ufpb.br/rbse/HartleyArt.pdf

Hartling, L., Lindner, E., Spalthoff, U., & Britton, M. (2013). Humiliation: A nuclear bomb of emotions? *Psicología Política, 46*, 55–76. Retrieved from http://www.uv.es/garzon/psicologia%20politica/N46-3.pdf

Hove, M., Ngwerume, E., & Muchemwa, C. (2013). The urban crisis in sub-Saharan Africa: A threat to human security and sustainable development. *Stability – International Journal of Security and Development, 2*(1). doi:http://doi.org/10.5334/sta.ap.

Hunter, P. R., & Fewtrell, L. (2001). Acceptable risk. In L. Fewtrell, & J. Bartram (Eds.), *Water quality: Guidelines, standards and health.* London: IWA Publishing. Integrated Regional Information Networks. (2008). *Kenya: Separated children eking a living in a Rift Valley town.* Retrieved from Integrated Regional Information Networks website: www.irinnews.org/Report/80267/KENYA-separated-children-eking-a-living-in-Rift-valley-town

Integrated Regional Information Networks. (2013, December 4). The hidden crisis in urban slums. *ReliefWeb.* Retrieved from http://reliefweb.int/report/kenya/hidden-crisis-urban-slums

International Organization for Migration (IOM). (2011). *Integrated biological and behavioural surveillance survey among migrant female sex workers in Nairobi, Kenya 2010. Healthy migrants in healthy communities.* Retrieved from the International Organization for Migration website: http://health.iom.int/

Joint United Nations Programme on HIV/AIDS (UNAIDS). (2008, May). *Facts about HIV.* Retrieved from http://data.unaids.org/pub/FactSheet/2008/20080519_fastfacts_hiv_en.pdf.

Joint United Nations Programme on HIV/AIDS (UNAIDS). (2011b). A New Investment Framework for the Global HIV Response. (UNAIDS Issues Brief). Geneva: UNAIDS.

Joint United Nations Programme on HIV/AIDS (UNAIDS). (2014a). *UNAIDS briefing book July 2014.* Geneva: UNAIDS.

Joint United Nations Programme on HIV/AIDS (UNAIDS). (2014b). *The gap report.* Geneva: UNAIDS.

Joint United Nations Programme on HIV/AIDS (UNAIDS). (2014c). *The cities report.* Retrieved from http://issuu.com/pm.dstaids.sp/docs/jc2687_thecitiesreport_en

Joint United Nations Programme on HIV/AIDS (UNAIDS). (2015). Leaders from around the world are All In to end the AIDS epidemic among adolescents. *Press Release.* Retrieved from http://www.unaids.org/en/resources/presscentre/pressreleaseandstatementarchive/2015/february/20150217_PR_all-in

Jorgenson, A. K., & Rice, J. (2012). Urban Slums and Children's Health. In Karides, F. A. (Ed.) Journal of World-Systems Research, 18(1), 103-116. Retrieved from http://www.jwsr.org/wp-content/uploads/2013/02/jorgenson rice-vol18n1.pdf.

Kahneman, D. K., & Krueger, A. B. (2006). Developments in the measurements of subjective well-being. *The Journal of Economic Perspectives, 20*(1), 3–24. doi:10.1257/089533006776526030.

Kenya National AIDS & STI Control Programme (NASCOP) & Ministry of Health. (2013). Kenya most at risk population size estimate consensus, 2012/2013. Nairobi: Kenya National AIDS & STI Control Programme (NASCOP)

King, R. (1999). *Sexual behavior change for HIV: Where have theories taken us?* (Key Material No. UNAIDS/99.27E). Retrieved from http://www.popline.org/node/533607#sthash.KICxIgul.dpuf

Lamba, D. (1994). The forgotten half; environmental health in Nairobi's poverty areas. *Environment and Urbanization, 6*, 164–168.

Lever, S. (2010, May 30). *Personal resilience.* Retrieved from Sally Lever website: http://www.sallylever.co.uk

Lindner, E. (2006). *Making enemies. Humiliation and international conflict.* Westport/London: Greenwood/Praeger Security International.

Lindner, E. (2009). *Emotion and conflict: How human rights can dignify emotion and help us wage good conflict.* Westport/London: Praeger.

Lindner, E. (2010). *Gender, humiliation and global security, dignifying relationships from love, sex, and parenthood to world affairs.* Santa Barbara: Prager Security International.

Lindner, E. (2012). *A dignity economy: Creating an economy that serves human dignity and preserves our planet.* Oslo: Dignity Press.

Ludi, E., & Bird, K. (2007, September). *Risks & vulnerability* (Brief No 3). Retrieved from http://www.odi.org/sites/odi.org.uk/files/odi-assets/publications-opinion-files/5680.pdf

Madise, N. J., Ziraba, A. K., Inungu, J., Khamadi, S. A., Ezeh, A., Zulu, E. M., Kebaso, J., Okoth, V., & Mwau, M. (2012). Are slum dwellers at heightened risk of HIV infection than other urban residents? Evidence from population-based HIV prevalence surveys in Kenya. *Health & Place, 18*(5), 1144–1152. doi:10.1016/j.healthplace.2012.04.003.

Mberu, B. U. (2012, November 11). *Adolescent sexual and reproductive health and rights: Research evidence from sub-Saharan Africa.* PPD conference "Evidence for action: South-south collaboration for ICPD beyond 2014," Ruposhi Bangla Hotel, Dhaka. Abstract retrieved from http://r4d.dfid.gov.uk/PDF/Outputs/StepUp/2012_PPDMberu.pdf

McLeish, K. (1993). *Bloomsbury guide to human thought.* London: Bloomsbury Publications.

McLeroy, K. R., Bibeau, D., Steckler, A., & Glanz, K. (1988). An ecological perspective on health promotion programs. *Health Education Quarterly, 15*(4), 351–377. Retrieved from http://www.ncbi.nlm.nih.gov/pubmed/3068205

Ministry of Health, Kenya (2012). *Kenya HIV Estimates.* Nairobi: Ministry of Health

Nairobi City Council/County Health Services. (2014). Nairobi city county response to the HIV epidemic. Unpublished raw data.

Oxford Dictionaries. (2015). Oxford University Press. Retrieved from http://www.oxforddictionaries.com/definition/english/dignity

Pamoja Trust. (2009). *An inventory of the slums in Nairobi.* Nairobi: Matrix Consultants.

Power, M. (2013, June 20). *Why no one is immune to HIV and why I was wrong.* Retrieved from http://mylespower.co.uk/2013/06/20/5125/

Shultziner, D., & Rabinovici, I. (2011). Human dignity, self-worth and humiliation: A comparative legal-psychological approach. *Psychology, Public Policy, and Law, 18*(1). doi:http://dx.doi.org/10.2139/ssrn.1964371.

Sifiris, D., & Myhre, J. (2015, June 5). Prevalence/incidence – Definition – HIV/AIDS. *About Health.* Retrieved from http://aids.about.com/od/hivaidsletteri/g/Prevalence-incidence-glosary-defination.htm

Smith, D. A. (1987). Overurbanization reconceptualized: A political economy of the world- systems approach. *Urban Affairs Quarterly, 23*(2), 270–294. doi:10.1177/004208168702300206 4.

Sommers, M. (2011). Governance, security and culture. Assessing Africa's youth bulge. *International Journal of Conflict and Violence, 5*(2), 292–303. Retrieved from http://www.academia.edu/5689491/Governance_Security_and_Culture_Assessing_Africa_s_Youth_Bulge

Sudan Tribune. (2014, June 2). South Sudan: HIV infection rates rising in central equatoria, officials say. *allAfrica.* Retrieved from http://allafrica.com/stories/201406090800.html

Sweat, M., & Denison, J. (1995). Reducing HIV incidence in developing countries with structural and environmental interventions. *AIDS, 9*(Suppl A), 251–257. Retrieved from https://www.researchgate.net/publication/14384926_Sweat_M.D.__Denison_J.A._Reducing_HIV_incidence_in_developing_countries_with_structural_and_environmental_interventions._AIDS_9_S251-S257

The Little Oxford Dictionary. (1998). Oxford: Oxford University Press.

United Nation Human Rights Office of the High Commissioner for Human Rights (UNOHCHR) (1989). *Convention on the Rights of the Child.* Retrieved from http://www.ohchr.org/EN/ProfessionalInterest/Pages/CRC.aspx.

United Nations. (2014, July 10). *World's population increasingly urban with more than half living in urban areas.* Retrieved from http://www.un.org/en/development/desa/news/population/world-urbanization-prospects-2014.html

United Nations Children's Fund (UNICEF). (2012). *State of the world's children. Children in an urban world.* Retrieved from http://www.unicef.org/sowc2012/

United Nations Fund Population Fund (UNFPA). (2007). *State of world population 2007: Unleashing the potential of urban growth.* Retrieved from www.unfpa.org

United Nations Human Settlements Programme (UN–Habitat). (2005). *Kenya: Nairobi urban profile, regional urban sector profile study.* Nairobi: UN-Habitat.

United Nations Human Settlements Programme (UN–Habitat). (2006a). *Nairobi: Urban sector profile.* Retrieved from http://unhabitat.org/

United Nations Human Settlements Programme (UN–Habitat). (2006b). *State of the world's cities 2006/7. Human settlements programme: The millenium development goals and urban sustainability-30 years of shaping the Habitat agenda.* Retrieved from http://www.amazon.com/State-Worlds-Cities-2006-Sustainability/dp/1844073785

United Nations Human Settlements Programme (UN–Habitat). (2007). *Enhancing urban safety and security. Global report on human settlements.* Retrieved from http://unhabitat.org/

United Nations Human Settlements Programme (UN–Habitat). (2011). *23rd Governing Council of UN-Habitat.* Retrieved from http://unhabitat.org/

United Nations Human Settlements Programme (UN–Habitat). (2014a, May 14). *Harnessing the dual global trends of urbanization and the demographic youth bulge* (Issues Paper). Retrieved from http://www.un.org/en/ecosoc/julyhls/pdf13/hls_issue_note_un_habitat.pdf

United Nations Human Settlements Programme (UN–Habitat). (2014b). *CEB high-level committee on programmes. Twenty-seventh session.* Retrieved from http://unhabitat.org/

United Nations Office for Disaster Risk Reduction (UNISDR). (2012). *The 10 essentials for making cities resilient.* Retrieved from http://www.unisdr.org/campaign/resilientcities/toolkit/essentials

United Nations Office for Disaster Risk Reduction (UNISDR). (2014) *Urban risk reduction and resilience.* Retrieved from www.unisdr.org

United Nations Office for the Coordination of Humanitarian Affairs (UN/OCHA). (2015). *Kenya humanitarian overview.* Retrieved from https://fts.unocha.org/pageloader.aspx?page=emerg-emergencyCountryDetails&cc=ken

United States Agency for International Development (USAID). (2012). *Programmatic Guidance for reducing HIV and key population stigma and discrimination. Lao PDR and Myanmar.* Retrieved from http://www.healthpolicyinitiative.com/publications/documents/1509_1_SD_guidance_documents_9_27_12.pdf

United States Department of Health and Human Services. (2002). *Physical activity evaluation handbook.* Atlanta: US Department of Health and Human Services, Centers for Disease Control and Prevention.

Vlahov, D., Freudenberg, N., Proietti, F., Ompad, D., Quinn, A., Nandi, V., & Galea, S. (2007). Urban as a determinant of health. *Journal of Urban Health: Bulletin of the New York Academy of Medicine, 84*(1). doi:10.1007/s11524-007-9169-3.

World Bank. (2015). *OVC toolkit.* Retrieved from http://info.worldbank.org/etools/docs/library/162495/howknow/definitions.htm

World Health Organisation (WHO) & United Nations Human Settlements Programme (UN–Habitat). (2010). *Hidden cities unmasking and overcoming health inequities in urban settings.* Retrieved from http://www.who.int/kobe_centre/publications/hiddencities_media/who_un_habitat_hidden_cities_web.pdf?ua=1

Chapter 2
Vulnerability and Risk: Health and Wellbeing in the Slum

Abstract This chapter provides a synthesis of the major literature concerning human rights, health and wellbeing and, especially, sexual and reproductive health among young people in a rapidly urbanising world. Key aspects relating to the structural determinants of health in urban slum settings and the major theories which have sought to explain it are described.

Keywords Urban health • Human rights • Poverty • Housing insecurity • Violence • Marginalisation • Sexual and reproductive health • Adolescents • Structural determinants • Vulnerability • Risk • Resilience • Dignity and humiliation • Kenya

Health Care and Wellness: Perception and Assumptions

The literature presents a series of assumptions concerning young people and health care in the urban slum. However, the point of departure is very often the provision of physical health infrastructure and less so on questions of access and perceptions of its efficacy by the intended users towards formal health care. Although the multisectoral nature of HIV is widely accepted, no less so is the belief that it is first and foremost a health concern. There still remains an implicit assumption that promotion of health care by service providers will be largely understood for its inherent value by the target population (Fineman 2008; Kahneman and Krueger 2006). However, this assumption is not always borne out by the evidence. Chambers (1995), for example, pointed out that often multiple realities exist between development (health) professionals and the end user with each party drawing on a discreet frame of reference and value system. The world view of many young people, in which health care is made intelligible, is not widely understood or integrated into mainstream health messaging, nor is the process of how different age groups of young people prioritise needs directly relating to a complete sense of wellbeing (WHO 2012). The multidimensional nature of seeking and sustaining health and

© The Author 2016   15
G. Jones, *HIV and Young People: Risk and Resilience in the Urban Slum*,
SpringerBriefs in Public Health, DOI 10.1007/978-3-319-26814-9_2

wellness is rarely captured in the literature, and particularly so in the African slum environment. While informed mostly by studies on non-compliance to treatment regimens, which often assert the subject's role in managing illness and creating a sense of autonomy, the evidence remains wanting and especially in regard to personal choice, of purposeful behaviour and notably so along gender lines. Nowhere is this more apparent than in the case of young migrants' perception of accessing health care in urban settings which can seem bewildering if not intimidating (IOM 2011b). Seasonal migrants may avoid seeking health care owing to a fear of ridicule and debasement, a perception that has been shown among people living with HIV and their relationships with health-care providers (UNAIDS 2014b). The end result may be feelings of humiliation and, in turn, heightened vulnerability through risky behaviour choice.

Young people, between the ages of 12–24, are not a homogenous group. Arguably, the most profound differences appear in the age groups: 0–14 (children) and 15–24 (youth) (World Bank 2015b). Perceptions towards health care differ between the different age groups. Whereas there is much overlap between these cohorts, influenced largely by place and context, distinctions are still discernible in regard to physical and psychosocial development and a sense of place in the world (UNFPA 2014). Based on evidence drawn from a study in Nairobi's slums, the evidence also suggests that adolescents across different age cohorts, while being increasingly savvy about their own sexuality, are less aware of their sexual and reproductive health needs and the holistic nature of 'wellness' (APHRC 2014). Further and more detailed research is necessary to explain the differences in perception of good health among and between the age groups classified as 'young' (WHO and UN-Habitat 2010). Concerning sexual and reproductive health, service provision is skewed towards older groups of adolescents (Dick 2013), which in part is influenced by prevailing moral codes and ideas of acceptable behaviour. The lack of empirical evidence regarding young adolescents is striking given, for example, the absolute number of teenage pregnancies in slum dwellings (UNFPA 2003). One study in Nairobi's slums showed that pregnancies among young adolescent women still count for a significant percentage of urban fertility (Mumah et al. 2014). The lack of study on perception and assumption among child-bearing youth in which the holistic nature of health and personal security is made explicit still presents itself as a significant gap.

A number of recurring themes concerning young people's perception of living in a modern urban slum appear in the research. What emerges is a commonality or pattern in regard to perceiving threat and choices of individual and collective response. These perceptions provide the fabric on which subsequent decisions are made, that interpret and make sense of the structural determinants of a life lived, for many slum-dwellers, in harsh and relentless conditions. The evidence, however, needs expanding when it comes to questions of how subjective experience gained in the social sphere leads to the choices made by slum-dwelling youth which can often put at immediate risk personal health and wellbeing. At the centre of this discussion of perception is the individual's sense of self, status and standing in the community.

There is a gap in the literature regarding the relationship between health, poverty, powerlessness and experiences of disempowerment and humiliation. Much of the research to date has not challenged the tendency to regard these experiences as largely separate in considerations of health and wellness. Moreover, the dynamic and evolving nature of subjective perception of humiliation and dignity and the place of structural determinants remains missing from current empirical evidence (Lindner 2012). This is striking given that 'dignity', however defined, is the core premise on which all universal health care proceeds (WHO 2006). It is argued that only through a composite analysis of the subjective experience of violence, poverty and social exclusion can the pathogenesis of psychosocial disorders associated with urban slum existence be truly understood (Hartling et al. 2013; Lindner 2010). Such enquiry would help, inter alia, to strengthen an understanding of how perceptions of vulnerability are constructed, change and become manifested in certain patterns of behaviour.

In an examination of health and rights, Leidner et al. (2012) demonstrated an association between subjective feelings of powerlessness and that of anger, shame and humiliation. Given its purported impact on negative interpersonal and inter-group behaviours and role in helping to shape social life, empirical research on humiliation in all settings is lacking, in particular, the outcome of repeated experiences of humiliation. As Leidner et al. (2012) also found, humiliation has a direct bearing on difficulties relating to learning and educational achievement, disorders related to trauma, impoverishment and intergroup violence and conflict. APHRC (2014) demonstrated in its longitudinal study of Nairobi's slums that the most vulnerable populations to ill health are those with the lowest levels of education and with a history of violence and incarceration. It is held that in any situation of powerlessness, there is an asymmetry between the 'humiliator' and 'humiliatee' in which the latter is more vulnerable and often dependent on the former. There are in effect multiple realities and divergent perceptions premised on notions of power and knowledge. The relevance of this assertion to the relationship between health-care provider and user of the service requires substantiating through further study. The assumption that this relationship is neutral, however, is becoming increasingly contested in the literature and notably in the case of recently arrived HIV-positive migrants into alien urban neighbourhoods.

Health and Human Rights: An Urban Perspective

Health is at the heart of the international urban development agenda and articulated through the Millennium Development Goals (MDGs),[1] founded on the principle of human rights and the right to health for all. This right to health underpins a dignified

---

[1] 'The Millennium Development Goals (MDGs) are eight goals to be achieved by 2015 that respond to the world's main development challenges. The MDGs were established in the Millennium Declaration that was adopted by 189 nations-and signed by 147 heads of state and governments during the UN Millennium Summit in September 2000' (Basic Education Coalition 2015). Three of the eight MDGs, eight of the 18 MDG targets and 18 of the 48 MDG indicators of progress are health related.

life. Moreover, in its interpretation, each factor relating to obtaining and maintaining sound health is considered equally important.[2] It is claimed that there is notable progress in drawing global attention to the principle of acceptable levels of health for all and in which resources for addressing bottlenecks in service provision have been revitalised (Basic Education Coalition 2015). But in a rapidly urbanising world, health care for all remains an elusive target, as patterns of sickness and disease evolve and are increasingly impacted by the natural and social environment (Kjellstrom et al. 2007). David et al. (2007) claims that basic principles of the public health system are challenged in the modern urban environment, largely owing to the fact that cities constantly evolve and are inherently dynamic. To effectively control infectious disease, notably HIV, tuberculosis and vector-borne agents, fundamental changes are called for so that those who are hardest to reach but have the greatest health needs can still realise their right to the best possible health care (David et al. 2007). Long-standing assumptions in health care and related provision in resource-constrained environments defined by structural disempowerment have to be identified by research, especially in the wake of HIV, social prejudice and their cumulative impact on feelings of wellbeing and health status. As the 'social determinants of disease model' helps explain, the current practice of targeting and prioritising health interventions, no matter how precise the aim, will have little hope of obtaining and sustaining 'health rights' until the deep inequities in accessing health care for the urban poor are addressed (David et al. 2007).

The relationship between sickness, care and cure and achieving a sense of wellbeing and universal health for all is, as it always has been, contentious and continuous to be explained by an array of social theories. In a study of children's wellbeing in the urban slum, Jorgenson and Rice (2012) make the case that in this maelstrom of communicable and non-communicable disease, it is rarely a straightforward path from sickness to sustainable health. In an environment where accessing resources are largely defined by power relations, Lindner (2012) states that realising human rights and promoting a life of dignity and health will always remain problematic. This perspective is at the heart of much socio-economic analysis as to who benefits from the gamut of scientific advance for the prevention and treatment of HIV (Cleary et al. 2012). Even with the advent of life-saving ART, in eastern and southern Africa, treatment coverage is only at 37 per cent among all people living with HIV (UNAIDS 2014a).[3] The evidence strongly suggests that a shift in the sociopolitical dynamics that determine access and availability remains the cornerstone for ending AIDS.

---

[2] The 1946 Constitution of the World Health Organization (WHO) preamble defines health as 'a state of complete physical, mental and social well-being and not merely the absence of disease or infirmity' and that 'the enjoyment of the highest attainable standard of health is one of the fundamental rights of every human being without distinction of race, religion, political belief, economic or social condition'.

[3] 'Standard antiretroviral therapy (ART) consists of the combination of at least three antiretroviral (ARV) drugs to maximally suppress the HIV virus and stop the progression of HIV disease' (WHO 2015).

In assessing the situation across the subcontinent, the African Union (2013a) highlighted the continuing plight of vulnerable women and adolescents and urged governments to see the link between poverty, health, peace and security. Further, the emerging priority is identified as the need to better understand the connection of HIV with women and children's vulnerability in relation to sexual and reproductive health in the context of civil conflict and the urban slum[4] (African Union 2013b). In a resource-constrained environment and one in which civil conflict so often prevails, the question remains, however, on the status of recent and current action within urban poor communities and taking any successful intervention to scale (African Union 2013a). However, empirical data arguably points to only modest achievement across the continent. The literature increasingly points to a re-evaluation of conventional approaches in policy and public health in reducing vulnerability by more fully understanding the nature and nuances of vulnerability and the matter of 'right of access' for all slum-dwelling populations.

The interrelationship between health and the language of human rights is widely recognised, notably, in the correlation between poverty, poor health and, inter alia, shorter life spans (Isunju et al. 2011). Glaeser et al. (2008) point to the global phenomenon of rapid urbanisation and the 'urbanisation of poverty' in much of the developing world. By perforce, this means that public health policy must fundamentally shift to better address emerging trends in burgeoning urban centres. Rights and access are never static but dynamic and diverse. Based on a broad range of indicators, it is claimed that urban poverty is becoming feminised with poor urban women and their dependents at considerably higher risk for multiple health concerns (Chant 1997). The relationship between health and gender has long been noted (UNAIDS 2011b). Sexual and reproductive health is especially challenged in the poorest urban settings – urban slums – and that lack of progress on core indicators in urban contexts is fundamentally undermining progress in meeting national targets of health care and ultimately the MDGs (Mberu 2012). An undermining of sexual and reproductive health has immediate ramifications in the prevention of HIV and the right to health and life. The link between poor sexual and reproductive health services prioritising populations most heavily infected and affected by HIV and AIDS has been clearly established (UNFPA 2008).

Realising the basic human right to access the best possible level of health care, and then maintaining a healthy lifestyle, is as complex as it is problematic. Wilson (2009) argued that concerning the social determinants of health, the matter goes far beyond a matter of physical infrastructure, trained medical personnel and provision of resources and must look at other social and familial influences. For many slum residents, it has been argued, there never was the necessary nurturing or guidance in their formative years on how to obtain and then maintain a healthy lifestyle

---

[4] 'In its broadest sense, sexual and reproductive health includes: family planning; maternal and perinatal health; sexually transmitted and reproductive tract infections; and prevention of unsafe abortions' (WHO 2013).

(Wilson 2009). Subjective perceptions of health and wellbeing may well exist and that stands counterposed to the more conventional understandings of the term. What measure to use, and what voice to listen to in deciding on matters of wellbeing and the realisation of health rights, according to WHO (2003) remains the subject of much debate. Enduring attitudes and habitual behaviour patterns may undermine attempts at obtaining the best possible level of health and be rooted in simply not knowing what alternatives exist (Wilson 2009). Messages concerning the practice of good health can be interpreted in multiple ways and evaluated for their relevance depending on background, personal circumstance and experience (Springer et al. 2003). The message of rights is far from straightforward and involves layers of interpretation by significant others which for children is very often through primary care givers.

On a daily basis, the urban poor face a range of health hazards related to a complex mix of physical, social and economic determinants (UN-Habitat 2013b). Dealing constantly with these hazards and unable to affect any form of meaningful change are in themselves manifestations of disempowerment and an overarching alienation from decision-making processes (Lindner 2010). According to UN-Habitat (2013a), the reality for slum-dwellers demonstrates that people living in poverty are trapped in their present situation and excluded from the rest of the society; for them, the luxury of choice simply does not exist. Routinely disempowered and disenfranchised, the urban poor are consistently challenged in building resilient communities (Mutisya 2010; United Nations Population Division 1998). This situation sits directly at odds with a 'rights-based' approach which emphasises the need for civic engagement and having the option to take a position in matters directly relating to one's health and wellbeing (United Nations Development Programme (UNDP) 2012a).

The literature has shown how many migrant populations can be at particular risk of not accessing basic health care. For them, the situation is compounded by numerous sociopolitical factors that may not improve in the long term (IOM 2011b). Leidner et al. (2012) found that feelings of humiliation as experienced through association with a particular group can be profound and work against realising even the most basic of health rights. The relevance to marginalised populations living with a constant threat of abuse, including physical harm, is immediate as it is far reaching. Yet there is a dearth of research in the literature on this subjective experience, especially as played out in the urban slum among concentrations of migrant and ethnic minorities (Mberu et al. 2014). The means to avoid experiencing humiliation are manifold as they are complex and lie at the heart of personal and collective resilience (Lindner 2012).

The case for 'health rights' in the urban slums is made clear by comprehensive global research. That is, squalid living conditions, lack of access to essential services, unsafe and insecure living conditions combined with material deprivation impacting on health and wellbeing. David et al. (2007) argue that owing to demonstrable levels of extreme poverty, informal settlements provide the 'worst-case' outcomes of the social determinants of health leaving its inhabitants wholly vulnerable to HIV/AIDS, tuberculosis and vector-borne diseases.

The Dynamics of Health, Poverty and Vulnerability: Housing, Security and Wellbeing in Slum Settings

In discussions of the structural determinants promoting or impeding access to health and rights, factors relating to housing and security are repeatedly shown in the literature as critical in shaping vulnerability, risk and resilience. They are each cornerstones of the most basic and fundamental building blocks of a system that integrates and is premised upon human rights. Whereas critical aspects of housing, security and wellbeing are often highlighted by health professionals, there is little evidence to show the development of alternative service delivery models more suited to meeting the demands of changing urban slum life. The implicit assumption appears that despite the challenges, which rarely include the relationship between provider (with power) and end user (powerless) in (resource-constrained) formal health settings, uptake of health services and desire for healthy lifestyles are absolute positions and, therefore, in much of the discourse, beyond questioning.

As Dugan (2011) states, a most basic health right directly relates to being able to live in a safe and secure environment. As this review shows, the interplay of housing instability and insecurity for many in the urban slum diminish the likelihood of seeing much practical application of these rights as well as the capacity to significantly reduce vulnerability by finding ways to manage the risk of ill health, including HIV infection. Proponents of human dignity and humiliation studies cite the poverty of suboptimum housing and violence, in all its forms, as having a profound influence on increasing vulnerability at an individual and collective level (Hartling et al. 2013).

Housing Insecurity and Notions of Social Cohesion

Housing is a most basic of human rights (UN-Habitat 2011). Housing in slums is often characterised by high population density, poor sanitation and in neighbourhoods with high rates of reported crime. These living conditions are directly connected to a range of health hazards, including a far greater likelihood of disease transmission, risky behaviours, physical injury and all forms of domestic and sexual violence (UN-Habitat 2010). The literature broadly agrees that vulnerability and risk are often rooted in suboptimal living conditions. Part of the vulnerability associated with slum residence stems from insecurity of tenure[5] as without this most basic security, there are substantial obstacles in planning and prioritising health care (Durand-Lasserve and Selod 2009). There is no standard definition in the literature

---

[5] UN-Habitat (2015) defines security of tenure as 'the right of all individuals and groups to effective protection against forced evictions. This right is enshrined in various declarations – including the Universal Declaration of Human Rights, the international Covenant on Economic, Social and Cultural Rights, the International Covenant on Civil and Political Rights, the Convention on the Elimination of all forms of Discrimination Against Women, the Covenant on the Elimination of All forms of Racial Discrimination and the Convention on the Rights of the Child' (UN-Habitat 2015).

as to what actually constitutes housing instability and homelessness applicable across culture and location (Vijayaraghavan et al. 2013). Moreover, conventional terminology is left wanting in describing the situation pertaining to the modern urban slum.[6] Global evidence has shown that recurring housing instability is a precursor to homelessness, which, in turn, majorly affects health and wellness (Kushel et al. 2006). Urban housing instability is a growing health concern worldwide; the lack of low-cost housing is seen as a major cause for increasing accounts of homelessness among the urban poor (UN- Habitat 2010). Both short- and long-term housing is a core component of the psychosocial risk factors associated with homelessness (Vijayaraghavan et al. 2013). The social and environmental stressors of poverty are key determinants for hypertension and premature mortality from illnesses, especially, cardiovascular disease (The American College of Obstetricians and Gynaecologists 2013). However, the absence of research specifically on the impact of humiliation and its dynamic relationship with the psychosocial dimensions of homelessness and the management of health and personal security in slums relevant to the developing world is significant, especially given the pervasiveness and routine nature of housing insecurity for so many of the urban poor.

Insight is provided by research carried out in low-costing housing urban settings in North America by Scott-Storey et al. (2009) that documents the social and economic stressors of living in extreme poverty as including poor neighbourhood conditions, lack of job security, constant threat of homelessness, interpersonal conflict and incarceration. Homeless women who have survived episodes of intimate partner violence, especially with a past history of being abused sexually or physically, are shown to be more likely to suffer hypertension than other social groups (Scott-Storey et al. 2009).

The evidence demonstrates a gender dynamic in the connection between poor health, housing instability and homelessness. The American College of Obstetricians and Gynaecologists (2013) recorded that homeless women faced a constant threat of injury and illness and regularly failed to seek necessary health care. Again, drawing on examples from poor urban neighbourhoods in North America, research similarly demonstrates that being homeless has a negative effect on all aspects of an individual's health, which includes the right to medical care. In response to chronic illness, homeless persons very often see the emergency department at major referral hospitals as the primary source of health care, and in the absence of preventive care, sickness and disease are very often presented at an advanced stage requiring longer hospitalisation (The American College of Obstetricians and Gynaecologists 2013). Teruya et al. (2010) noted that homeless women especially lacked preventive care especially regarding prenatal care and exhibited heightened rates of poor health status overall, including mental illness, poor birth outcomes and mortality. A close

---

[6] According to the National Alliance to End Homelessness, homelessness is defined as the state of an individual or family who lacks a fixed, regular and adequate night-time residence. Chronic homelessness is defined as 'an unaccompanied individual with a disabling condition who has either been continually homeless for a year or more or who has had at least four episodes of homelessness in the past three years' (The National Alliance to End Homelessness 2012).

connection between violence and homelessness among women has been demonstrated (The American College of Obstetricians and Gynaecologists 2013). The leading cause of homelessness for women (and dependents) in the North America is domestic and sexual violence, accounting for up to 50 per cent of all cases of homelessness (Jasinski et al. 2005). Based on a phenomenological study of homeless people carried out by Martins (2008), the major obstacles to health care are, firstly, social triaging; secondly, stigma for being homeless; thirdly, lack of care at all levels of the health system; fourthly, disrespectful treatment; and fifthly, feeling ignored by health-care providers. It has been argued that obstacles in accessing health care can lead to experiences of dehumanisation and debasement, key concepts in human dignity and humiliation studies (Lindner 2001). In the absence of empirical evidence, it is conjecture as to whether avoiding a shaming event is an act of self-protection and therefore an instance of self-affirming behaviour, even if in the long term it may result in failing health and wellbeing. By not having the information on homelessness in diverse settings in the urban slums of Africa leaves a notable gap in understanding the plight of the homeless and their attempts to dignify that life, which, at this stage, can only be assumed. The desire to dignify one's life, regardless of circumstance is, according to a broad spectrum of literature, a universal human trait.

With little security of tenure and the anxiety experienced from fear of losing house and home, risky behaviour, including 'risky sex'.[7] as well as 'medicating' through substance abuse, is recorded as providing a not uncommon means of escape (Parks 2014). Use of negative coping mechanisms is, in itself, an instance of resilience to persistent and multifarious hazards. However, these avenues of escape often lead to addiction and life-threatening obsession[8] in which resources dwindle and the situation exacerbates, calling on further use of the drug of choice and the cycle of dependence and destruction continues (Goodman and Hilton 2010).

Unsafe housing and homelessness are widely documented as increasing the risk of acquiring HIV (WHO and UN-Habitat 2010). There is a striking absence of research on how to avoid defaulting on antiretroviral therapy owing to unsafe and precarious housing conditions and following the rigours of a 'SMART' patient.[9] Adherence, for example, to an approved regimen of ART requires at least a modicum of safe storage in a reliable location (AIDSinfo 2014), a condition which can prove problematic in crowded and insecure living arrangements. Moreover, in these situations, there is a predictable lack of privacy in the safe keeping of ART

---

[7] Risky sex is behaviour that increases the risk of contracting sexually transmitted infections and experiencing unintended pregnancies. This behaviour includes: early sexual debut, multiple concurrent sexual partners, having sex under the influence of alcohol or drugs and unprotected sexual intercourse (webMD 2014).

[8] Addiction is defined as '…a persistent, compulsive dependence on a behaviour or substance; two types of addictions are noted: substance addictions (for example, alcoholism, drug abuse, and smoking); and process addictions (for example, gambling, spending, shopping, eating, and sexual activity)' (The Free Dictionary 2015).

[9] SMART is the: Strategies for the Management of Antiretroviral Therapy, in which treatment breaks are not recommended (Siegel and El-Sadr 2006).

medication. With high levels of stigma and discrimination, a strict confidentiality is often the only resource in treatment adherence and integration into the local community (AIDSinfo 2014). However, the need to 'keep secret' an HIV-positive status and treatment regimen can also lead to feelings of shame and resentment, which, in turn, militate against the principle of SMART practice as it may lead to situations in which treatment adherence becomes untenable. The evidence base on which to draw conclusive statements regarding storage, confidentiality and 'keeping appearances' in the local community, its overall effect on self-confidence, shame and social standing needs strengthening in all related research. The fact that there is arguably a dearth of critical enquiry can be taken as instance of one of the many implicit assumptions regarding treatment uptake and adherence. In the formulation of health policy, the assumption-cum-principle that slum-dwellers will always find ways and means to maintain a treatment regimen built on their own initiative remains under researched and creates a significant gap in the evidence.

In Kenya, millions of urban poor live with no security of tenure and face the prospect of homelessness (Pamoja 2009). This owes in large part to the systematic failure of officials to recognise the proliferation and reality of informal settlements and slums and to plan accordingly (Mutisya and Yarime 2011). By the end of 2010, more than 50,000 people were living alongside railway lines in Nairobi in makeshift dwellings and with the constant threat of forced eviction[10] (Amnesty International 2009). In the case of the informal settlement of Kibera, said to be home for up to a million people, the land is owned by the Kenya Railway Authorities with many dwellings considered as illegal and therefore not qualifying for social service provision (Ekdale 2011). In Nairobi's Mathare slum, residents faced threat of mass displacement and destruction of homes owing to the then city council's ideas of rehabilitating the area alongside the one water way running through the settlement (Amnesty International 2009). In the slums, business enterprise or 'structure owners' (Pamoja 2009) sees a profit in erecting dwellings for rent even though, for much of the settlement, there are no title deeds to the occupied land. In the case of illegal occupancy, there is little recourse to law enforcement from either side of the dispute (Pamoja 2009).

Large-scale displacement has taken place within the slum settlements of Nairobi (Kamungi 2013; Pamoja 2009). Mainly due to urban development policy, there are many examples of 'slum upgrading' along with construction of essential infrastructure such as road bypasses (Kamungi 2013). The Centre for Housing Rights and Evictions (2005) states that forced evictions are increasing and notably since 2001, due in part to the coming of a parliamentary democracy in Kenya (Metcalfe et al. 2011). Pamoja (2009) stated that in Nairobi, evictions have gone on without due process, consultation or compensation and involved excessive force or violence. With resources already stretched, the result is often catastrophic for impoverished people who lose home, assets and social networks, as well as access to water, work, health and education. As Mutisya and Yarime (2011) suggest, for many slum

---

[10] Forced eviction is the removal of people against their will from homes or land they occupy and in the absence of legal protection and safeguards (Amnesty International 2009).

inhabitants, the right to health and a dignified life is an aspirational goal with little practical relevance. The sense of powerlessness against structural determinants is overwhelming. Yet within this universe, slum residents dignify life and a lifestyle in line with a very particular, if not at times seemingly contradictory, value system that can reward, condone as well as condemn certain behaviour, including that relating to HIV and wilful transmission of the virus. Studies into urban subcultures and the value systems of young people – the largest group and cohort most infected and affected by HIV and AIDS – in Nairobi's slum require much further detailed research.

The reality of forced eviction, of involuntary migration, has immediate consequences for perceptions of powerlessness and inability to influence factors that majorly affect one's life. At a systemic level, insecure tenure institutionalises the social exclusion of the urban poor. A world view premised on feelings of hopelessness and marginalisation can quickly lead to feelings of despair and risky behaviour as well as an overall growing sense of vulnerability over which one has little control (Wilkinson and Marmot 2003; UN-Habitat 2012). Forced dislocation is a likely precursor for humiliation and subsequent ill health (Lindner 2001).

Yet in urban slum areas even with a history of social upheaval, another perspective emerges. Insecurity of house and home, however, does not necessarily mean an absence of community and social cohesion. Community action is well documented as a way of asserting human rights and has been seen in the literature as a form of resistance (Wilkinson and Marmot 2003). It is also a feature of collective resilience. A supportive and nurturing environment, it is held, can lead directly to positive health outcomes (WHO 2014). Social cohesion is an instance of asserting a sense of dignity and a protective mechanism against the fear of isolation and exclusion and can positively affect health and longevity (Wilkinson and Marmot 2003; Lindner 2009). Social cohesion, built on manifestations of trust, mutual obligation and respect, has an immediate effect on feelings of wellbeing and innovation (Lindner 2006). Social action stemming from a sense of community has been shown, for example, by young representatives from Nairobi's slums who have organised community-based responses to improve life and livelihoods (UNAIDS 2014c). A multitude of community partnerships, sometimes involving external actors, exist throughout Nairobi's slums which have supported collaborative initiatives aimed at promoting social organisation and enhance protection, education and microbusiness enterprise as well as improving the health status of its inhabitants, including HIV prevention and care (UN-Habitat 2007a).

In the same vein, this sense of belonging and personal status has been noted elsewhere including studies on the dynamics of peer groups identified with a clearly mapped urban territory that provide a sense of cohesion and order. Descriptive analysis often portrays the urban peer group in a negative light highlighting deviant subculture in which the membership seeks to assert its presence through overtly anti-social acts. For some theorists, deviancy is often the only option available for subpopulations largely disempowered and alienated from 'mainstream culture' (Brake 2013). The assertion of collective values can run roughshod over the health and wellbeing of the individual, and that the premise on which personal resilience is created becomes unsustainable. In studies on the sociology of deviance, the 'full social theory of deviance' drawing on neo-Marxist traditions has argued that these groups are often made up of individuals who have little hope of finding identity and achieving success through conformity to others' value systems (Thompson 2011).[11] This frustration can lead to violence and manifest in anti-social behaviour, directly played out in the immediate locality and within clearly marked boundaries and lines of physical separation between neighbourhoods. Social cohesion as evidenced here is proscribed and actively enforced, and not a matter of free will and voluntary participation.

The literature, however, has failed to conclusively explain how individuals aim to dignify their life through membership of a particular group or association in a particular area of the slum through engaging in acts contrary to understood notions of acceptable behaviour. As explained by the 'full social theory of deviance', violence is often one of the few ways in which the sense of frustration and anger from alienating structures can be expressed in the local neighbourhood and is a defining feature, especially for young males, of claiming social acceptance and dignifying life in a repressed society. Empirical evidence to support or refute this claim in the case of the urban African slum is wanting. However, the link between violence, subculture and HIV transmission is well documented.

Violence

Drawing on global experience, violence in cites is described as the other major defining feature shaping the vulnerability of urban slum-dwellers. A plethora of research has variously described slum environments as foci of violence and highlighted its impact on vulnerability to poor health outcomes among the urban poor (Sclar et al. 2005). The link between different forms of violence, notably sexual violence and acquisition of HIV, is long established (Fustos 2011). Moser (2004) argues that in addition to giving way to fear, exclusion and uncertainty, violence adversely affects the urban poor's ability to access vital resources to sustain life and livelihoods. This owes not only to the spatial, economic and social constraints posed by endemic violence but also the failure of the state to provide meaningful protection (Moser 2004).

According to Kyobutungi et al. (2008), most of the global criteria for violence at societal, community and individual levels apply in informal settlements. Criteria include lack of inhibition to perpetrate forms of violence, social disintegration, high residential instability and mobility, heterogeneous population density, absence of social cohesion, drug and alcohol abuse and limited employment opportunities. The manifestations of marginalisation of residents in slum-like settlements are inadequate service provision by social institutions, including functioning law

---

[11] Neo-Marxist approaches in the context of deviance studies have also been called 'radical criminology' (Thompson 2011).

enforcement. Perceived indifference by such institutions towards slum communities can result in community measures, chiefly, mob justice (Kyobutungi et al. 2008). Mob justice demonstrates self-defined notions of what is held to be true and the justification for enforcing this view, which, in effect, is the orchestration of the dominant and most powerful group's opinion within a community (Sekudu 2014). There was mob justice against men suspected of having same-sex relations in Kenya as a way to 'cleanse' the community of apparent evil (Human Rights Watch 2010). In Uganda, the country's penal code classifies homosexuality (and sex work) as 'crimes of morality' which led to forms of mob justice against minority groups (Porter 2014). Forms of mob justice have had their roots in xenophobic attacks in informal settlements in South Africa resulting in the destruction of homes and live-lihoods of migrants and non-local residents (Jaftha 2015). Documented in different parts and at different times in Nairobi's slums is the conspicuous absence of the rule of law and the existence of protection rackets as well as organised crime that create a climate of fear and intimidation (Kamungi 2013). According to Collazzoni et al. (2014), humiliation has helped perpetuate social tensions and led to different levels and forms of violence across social and geographic settings. Lindner (2009) further researched 'the need to conform' in order to avoid episodes of being seen as the outsider and fear of humiliation and ridicule in the public realm. Accounts of mea-sures taken to avoid the humiliation of being found to be HIV positive are docu-mented through numerous works on HIV stigma and discrimination (Williams 2014).

Research by Ziraba et al. (2011b) found that slum environments in Nairobi are pervasively unsafe and insecure. Looking at the causes and risk factors of fatal inju-ries in two slums in Nairobi, it was reported that intentional injuries accounted for some 51 per cent of all injuries (Ziraba et al. 2011b). Injuries due to personal vio-lence are the second leading contributor to mortality in Nairobi's slums (Kyobutungi et al. 2008). Violence is a key feature of slum life that contributes to persistent health burdens of the urban poor (Sclar et al. 2005). Research has demonstrated that vio-lence also plays an important role in the lives of young people living in slums. Moser (2004) reported that this violence has many physical and mental manifestations and has a direct bearing on behaviour and health, including child maltreatment, youth perpetrated violence, sexual- and gender-based violence and exploitation of less powerful social groups. The literature suggests that what is less researched is how violent acts help cement place and position within the African urban subculture and lead to a sense of wellbeing and particularly so for young people.

Young people, especially between the ages of 15 and 24, are at the centre of urban violence, both in terms of committing the largest number of violent acts and being the principle victims of violence (United Nations Office for Drugs and Crime (UNODC) 2012). Young people in Nairobi's slums are often victims of sexual vio-lence, including rape. Young people have reported that is not uncommon to be attacked at home or outside by peers, teachers, parents, family members, adult neighbours, romantic partners and strangers (Mumah et al. 2014). Street youth in particular are highly vulnerable to violence, abuse and HIV infection, noting, that it is this age cohort most infected and affected by HIV and AIDS.

Critical to a discussion of slum violence is that of gender-based violence which includes in its remit: sexual violence, domestic violence, intimate partner rape and intimate partner violence, all of which are identified as potential modes of transmitting HIV (Anderson et al. 2008).[12] Research conducted by Oduro et al. (2012) adopting a 'social ecological' approach highlighted how GBV is experienced by the subject and used by the perpetrator. In a study carried out in Ghana, Kenya and South Africa on the manifestations of gender-based violence, Oduro et al. (2012) made clear the critical links between school, community, street and family and the interplay of poverty with both macro- and microsystems of power contextualised by structural violence. Key to understanding the nuances of gender-based violence is the subjective experience of young people in the slum environment, characterised by limitation and constraint. In reinforcing collective notions of masculinity in the urban slum, men used violence against women as an expression of revenge and/or retribution, as a means to gain respect and to exercise control over female sexuality (Oduro et al. 2012). Oduro et al. (2012) saw this violence as essentially a result of living in abject poverty and a fundamental denial, especially for young people, of human rights. Slum-dwelling young women possibly motivated by the fear of humiliation have similarly been documented as perpetrators of violence towards women of similar age and background (Oduro et al. 2012).

Migrants to the city, and in particular involuntary migrants, may have fled situations of conflict and violence and carry trauma which, from what is known, largely goes untreated or recognised (IOM 2011a). Globally, the number of people displaced by conflict and violence has significantly increased (Lederer 2011). By the end of 2010, across 20 countries, almost three million people had been uprooted as a result of conflict and violence and over one million of these were in Africa (Lederer 2011). For these refugees and internally displaced people – all them involuntary migrants – many have faced repeated episodes of violence and conflict including killings, rape, torture and hunger and continue to suffer the effects of these experiences (Miller and Rasmussen 2010). Migration-associated stressors have been strongly identified with people fleeing persecution and violence (Miller and Rasmussen 2010). It is likely that these reported that these stressors build on pre-existing vulnerabilities and place the migrant at especial risk particularly with long-time urban residents in places of exile.

Research contests the exact relationship between situations of violent conflict and HIV. What is largely agreed is that the dynamics of HIV and AIDS is played out according to context (Porter 2014). The evidence suggests a higher risk of HIV transmission in post conflict settings, in part owing to greater mobility between areas of high and low HIV prevalence (Porter 2014). Following the upheaval experienced during the post-election violence of 2007/2008 in Kenya and the large-scale intra-urban and rural to urban displacement, Nairobi's slums became and remain effectively 'societies in transition' (Porter 2014).

---

[12] Gender-based violence refers to expectations and positions relating to social status based on gender which are in conflict with accepted modes of gender behaviour.

Evidence is lacking as to whether having had a prior experience of violence can help prepare the newly arrived migrant in the slum or conversely acts as an extra weight to carry. Processing and dealing with incidents of violence in large part is down to personal traits, an inner resilience or a sense of resignation to the inevitable (Lindner 2009). The adverse effects of extended periods of living with violence have been shown in bouts of depression and feelings of hopelessness and despair (McCord 1997). Caught in a spiral of violence and retaliation, the result is very often a continuing pattern of anti-social behaviour (Lindner 2009; McCord 1997).

Accessing Health Care in the Urban Slum: Structural Determinants and Cultural Practice

The literature demonstrates that the majority of slum-dwellers struggle to access basic health care and maintain healthy, non-threatening, lifestyles. As Shetty (2011) shows, for the majority of slum residents, health care is routinely unavailable and suboptimal. UNICEF (2012) reported that for the slum communities in Nairobi, health facilities were almost non-existent, with the vast majority of inhabitants relying on unregulated services of questionable quality invariably provided in run-down and poorly maintained clinics. UNICEF (2012) estimated that only 1 per cent of all health services utilised were public and accountable to health authorities. The conclusions drawn from the UNICEF report (2012) further corroborated the findings of a UN-Habitat account (2010) of the comprehensive lack of access to basic health services by people living in slums across Nairobi. From research conducted in different cities around the world, it appears that private pharmacies and, to a lesser extent, private clinics are often the predominant form of health care for slum inhabitants (Khan et al. 2012). These establishments are often managed by poorly qualified or inexperienced health-care providers offering unregulated services (Khan et al. 2012). As Unger and Riley (2007) state, in the private sector, fees and costs are always involved and at all stages of health care, which, for those living in extreme poverty, can seem prohibitive or be simply out of reach.

A study carried out in Namibia found that in urban slum neighbourhoods in Windhoek, the capital city, the highest recorded HIV incidence and prevalence were in areas with the lowest concentration of any form of health facility (UNAIDS 2013c). Similar situations are discernible in other African cities. The evidence suggests that slum communities are powerless to influence health-care provision from city authorities and/or not aware that it is their right to demand such services (UNDP 2012a).

Studies on Nairobi's slums find a range of factors contributing to poor health outcomes. Garenne (2010) found that in Nairobi's slums, increasing under five mortality was caused by a lack of potable water and a functioning system of sanitation, concentrations of different population groups, suboptimal housing, as well as low levels of nutrition, pervasive poverty, insecurity and violence and not being able to access even the most basic forms of preventive and therapeutic health care. Kyobutungi et al. (2008) noted that the urban poor in Nairobi fare worse than their rural counterparts on nearly all health indicators, with half of all deaths attributable to HIV and tuberculosis.[13] The poor health status of slum children has been explained by a continuous exposure to environmental hazards, lack of social services and minimal protection or guidance on how to stay healthy from primary care givers (Premji 2014). Research in diverse settings has shown that outdoor and indoor air pollution is a critical factor in children's poor health. Many slums are situated near industrial areas and road transport networks, and in slum dwellings most cooking is conducted indoors creating smoke which is dangerous to inhale, especially for young children (Cotton 2013). According to Egondi et al. (2013), air pollution in two of Nairobi's slums exceeded internationally accepted standards by a 100-fold and that residents were regularly exposed to life-threatening air pollutants including poisonous gases.

Within this context, slum-dwellers have little or no power and extremely limited resources to affect meaningful change in their circumstances, except for the worse. It follows that these residents experience heightened risk of acquiring HIV, tuberculosis and vector-borne diseases, owing to increased exposure to disease agents and infection (WHO 2010a). Caldwell (2014) argues that social inequities predispose slum-dwellers to infectious disease that limits options for dealing with sickness and disease and that economic marginalisation in the informal settlement, specifically the cost of health care, is the single greatest barrier for sustained wellness.

Turan and Besirli (2008) found that mental health in the slum is too often overlooked in discussions of wellbeing and social cohesion. Possibly due to the overriding need to provide for the basics of life – food, water and shelter – seeking help for mental health is, by and large, not considered a pressing necessity. Living every day in a world of violence and intimidation with constant noise, pollution, poor housing and overcrowding and in conditions of abject poverty and especially for migrant communities cultural dislocation can prove overwhelming. These conditions give way to feelings of depression, anxiety, fear and violence inwardly and outwardly directed (Turan and Besirli 2008).

Sexual and Reproductive Health in Urban Africa

Seeing the structural inequities at the core of poor health outcomes, some modest improvement in reproductive health policies and service delivery has been noted in sub-Saharan Africa (UNFPA 2014). However, the region has failed to demonstrate lasting change in addressing the reproductive health of slum residents, as the case of Nairobi city's slums demonstrates. Luke et al. (2012) found that slum settlements

---

[13] 'The risk of developing tuberculosis (TB) is estimated to be between 26 and 31 times greater in people living with HIV (PLHIV) than among those without HIV infection. In 2013, there were nine million new cases of TB of which 1.1 million were among PLHIV'. TB is consistently found in poorer populations (WHO 2015).

performed poorly on a number of key indicators concerning sexual and reproductive health compared to the average for the city of Nairobi, including fertility rates, child and infant mortality, disease prevalence, unemployment and poverty (APHRC 2002; Ziraba et al. 2009). Nairobi's slum residents also exhibit significant disadvantages likely to undermine reproductive health, with respect to living conditions, access to health services including family planning services, sexual violence and risky sexual practices (Fotso et al. 2008, 2009; Taffa et al. 2005).

A number of studies have looked at the connections between poverty, slum residence and sexual behaviour. Kamndaya et al. (2014) note that poverty is a key driver of sexual risk-taking behaviour in urban slums, and studies carried out in high-income countries have found a strong association between material deprivation and health behaviour (Greif 2012; Heflin and Iceland 2009). There is, however, debate on the applicability of modelling techniques developed in high-income countries and their relevance in low-income countries which consistently demonstrate a link between health, risk taking and material deprivation (Burns and Snow 2012). However, Greif (2012) conceptualised deprivation using local constructs of unmet basic needs of housing, health care and food and found a positive association with women's likelihood to engage in risky sexual behaviour, including sex work and multiple sexual partners in Nairobi's slums. The extent to which her findings can be extrapolated and compared to the experience of young men is still to be proven by research.

Greif (2012) strengthened the evidence of a link between slum residence, poverty, urbanisation and risky sex through a five city study in five different countries in Africa. A firm pattern of risky sex in slums was demonstrated in each of the five cities, compared with non-slum residence, based on indicators of early sexual debut, lower condom use and multiple sexual partners. Similarly, the work of Zulu et al. (2002) on urban poverty, slum residence and health outcomes documented the effect of slum residence on sexual behaviour in Nairobi and found that slum residents were consistently vulnerable to various reproductive health risks. Dodoo et al. (2007) looked into whether the disadvantage found by Zulu et al. (2011) was truly an urban poverty effect or simply one generally of poverty. Their comparison of rural and urban contexts reinforced the argument for a unique impact of urban poverty and adverse sexual outcomes. Multiple earlier studies have shown that local disadvantage can be a powerful predictor of risk associated with early sexual debut, low levels of contraceptive use and multiple concurrent sexual partners (Browing et al. 2005). Despite this plethora of information, much of the research has failed to fully discern, or only points to, the various value systems and socially constructed frames of reference which sanction acceptable and non-acceptable behaviour and subjective perception of how factors directly affecting life and livelihoods are ranked and interpreted. Arguably, there is a misplaced assumption in the literature that risky behaviour will hold the same meaning and import for slum-dwelling young people as it does for non-slum-dwelling young people as well as cadres of health professionals.

Ndugwa et al. (2011) found that living in urban slums limits women's ability to control their fertility and implement their fertility preferences. For example, in

Korogocho and Viwandani slums in Nairobi, research showed that almost half (47 per cent) of pregnancies are unwanted and/or unintended. Ziraba et al. (2009) report that maternal mortality rates in the urban slums are almost double the national average, with an estimated 706 maternal deaths for every 100,000 live births, compared to 488 per 100,000 live births for all Kenya. Studies indicate that these trends are found in urban slums in other African countries, with results the same or worse on standard indicators, notably child mortality (UN-Habitat 2003b). In their study of women, poverty and adverse maternal outcomes in Nairobi, Izugbara and Ngilangwa (2010) argue that for slum-dwelling women, there is an urgent need to better understand the holistic nature of maternal outcomes – including the role of men and dependants – and the link between women's livelihoods, health and overall wellbeing within a patriarchal society. The dominant practice in researching sexual and reproductive health in Nairobi's slums, however, has arguably lent towards a 'silo approach' and a focus on those aspects which are more conducive to quantifiable analysis. The evolving (sub-)cultural understanding of reproductive and sexual health among young urban slum-dwellers in Nairobi requires further focussed qualitative investigation.

Adolescent Sexual and Reproductive Health

Although little data is specific to slum-dwelling adolescents from migrant families, research on sexual and reproductive health in sub-Saharan Africa indicates that both resident and migrant young Africans have the worst indicators for reproductive health compared with the global picture, including age of sexual debut and contraceptive use (Okonofua 2007). A study conducted by Luke et al. (2012) notes that early sexual debut is highly associated with sexually transmitted infections, HIV, precancerous changes of the cervix, unwanted pregnancy and pregnancy complications. Furthermore, a high percentage of young women aged 15–19 have had sexual intercourse in a number of sub-Saharan African countries – 73 per cent in Liberia, 53 per cent in Nigeria, 49 per cent in Uganda and 32 per cent in Botswana (Mberu 2012). Orphans[14] and vulnerable children are especially vulnerable due to lack of social and economic support; in South Africa, 23 per cent of orphans reported having had sex by the age of 13, which stands in contrast to 15 per cent of non-orphans (Mberu 2012).

Early marriage and childbirth remain key challenges to sexual and reproductive health in the region. In the developing world, one in every three girls are married

---

[14] 'Commonly defined definitions of orphan and vulnerable children include: orphaned by the death of one or both parents; abandoned by parents; living in extreme poverty; living with a disability; affected by armed conflicts; abused by parents or their carers; malnourished due to extreme poverty; HIV-positive; marginalized, stigmatized or discriminated against. All vulnerable children have no reliable social safety networks to effectively manage the risks to which they are daily exposed' (Home Grown School Feeding 2015).

before the age of 18 and 1 in 9 are married before the age of 15 (International Centre for Research on Women (ICRW) 2015). Mberu (2012) reports that early marriage is still relatively common in sub-Saharan Africa, with at least one in six young women married before the age of 15 and with the mean age of brides at 15 years in Niger, 16.5 years in Cameroon and 17.5 years in Burkina Faso. There is also great age asymmetry among marital and sexual partners, reflecting the patriarchal nature of sub-Saharan Africa. Asymmetric partner age has been shown to be a key route for HIV transmission (Luke 2005). The mean age difference between husband and wife is 15 years in Cameroon and 7 years in Kenya (Barbieri and Hertrich 2005; Mberu 2012).

The significant proportion of young mothers within or outside a recognised marriage union with unwanted pregnancies is highlighted as a major aspect of vulnerability (Mberu 2012). In part owing to the unwanted nature of the pregnancy for many unmarried young slum-dwelling women in Nairobi aged 15–19, adolescents are more likely to resort to unsafe abortions with 57 per cent of all unsafe abortions annually occur among young women between the ages of 15–19 years (Kenya Human Rights Commission 2010; Mberu 2012).[15] Pregnant young women are also more likely to drop out of school: 13,000 Kenyan young women drop out of school annually owing to reasons directly related to pregnancy, and 13 per cent of young women drop out of school before completion in order to marry in which the immediate bearing of children is culturally expected (Luke et al. 2012; Mberu 2012). Status earned from child bearing and in particular experience gained from the burden of child responsibility has not been systematically covered by empirical enquiry, possibly owing to the often unspoken assumption that young child bearing is 'bad' regardless of context. Whereas mostly social anthropological study has shown the importance of child rearing in providing a sense of belonging and status, this work is largely carried out in rural settings, leaving a significant gap in regard to modern urban environments. The evidence requires substantiating as to whether child bearing in the slum while still young is generally perceived as a preferred option for enhancing standing in the local community as opposed to seeking formal education, not having children and traveling outside of the immediate location. This is especially so regarding the case for young migrant women newly arrived into the urban slum.

Kabiru (2015) report that sexual and reproductive health for young people is strongly influenced by competing priorities and principles. A number of factors impact on whether young people access related services that include unmarried status, discussing matters of a sexual nature, perceived attitudes of care providers, misconceptions regarding sexuality including forms of contraception and attitudes towards premarital sex. The gender imbalance in sexual decision-making influences teen women's contraceptive use; in a Malawi study, most adolescent young women said that it is easier to risk pregnancy than to ask their partner to use a condom (Tavory and Swidler 2009). WHO (2012) has stressed the urgency in generating more evidence on the needs and preferences of urban slum-dwelling young people and scaling up of evidence-informed delivery mechanisms, chief of which is

---

[15] An unsafe abortion is the termination of a pregnancy by people lacking the necessary skills, or in an environment lacking minimal medical standards, or both (Wikipedia 2015).

disaggregated and location specific information that expands current knowledge on the urban dynamics of adolescent sexual health.

The concept of sex as a social currency helps provide insight into the dynamic of sexual health for urban-based youth. In this regard, sex as a social currency draws on the entirety of actual and potential resources stemming from urban social networks that create the means to access information and knowledge as an integral part of the formation of identity, status and recognition (Dobransky 2015; Vilvadi 2010). Evidence for sex as a social currency in the modern urban slum requires further and comprehensive research. As such, until such evidence is generated, a key aspect in vulnerability remains inadequately addressed and notably so for most at risk populations. There appears little cross-cultural study on the question of personal and social gain through using sexual liaisons as a currency resource holding the opportunity for personal and familial advancement as well as cementing social standing in the local community (Dobransky 2015). Academic enquiry has largely concerned itself with related notions of 'social capital' and social networks and particularly in the context of migrant communities arriving in urban centres.

Social Marginalisation

The literature clearly shows that social marginalisation is a significant barrier to accessing health care. Many so-called marginalised populations concentrate in urban centres to facilitate social networking and because it offers a degree of protection (UNAIDS 2014c). These groups include men who have sex with men (MSM), people who inject drugs (PWID), sex workers (SW) and transgender people, all of whom have consistently have the highest rates of HIV anywhere in the world. Owing much to the deterrent effects of stigma, discrimination and social isolation, these groups are far less likely to access the full range of HIV services available at private and/or public health institutions (UNAIDS 2011b). For many, routine humiliation by health-care professionals is not uncommon. This fact is well documented. What is much less studied is how people from these marginalised groups seek to dignify their existence and the priority placed on achieving and maintaining sound health. Overall, their resilience largely goes unrecognised and undocumented.

Stigma has been described as an 'epidemic within an epidemic' (Plummer and McLean 2010). Stigma, sustained over time and across settings, can place already vulnerable people at further risk through shaming, exclusion and denial. According to Plummer and McLean (2010), stigma is experienced by concealing infection and driving it from the reach of health-care services. Stigma to HIV infection further deepens a sense of vulnerability and hurt, hinders support networks, leads to anti-social behaviour and ultimately weakens political will (Plummer and McLean 2010). The association between stigma and discrimination and humiliation and the cumulative effect on vulnerability and risky behaviour can only be assumed as the link, as yet, is to be fully proven.

Living with HIV has, from the outset, proved a source of stigma. UNAIDS (2014b) states that there is little hope of reducing HIV rates without significantly reducing levels of social stigma and discrimination. Socially stigmatising characteristics of the groups most afflicted by the epidemic serve to further emphasise HIV-related stigma that can give way to 'super-stigmatisation' in that exclusion, and the devaluation of people living with HIV (PLHIV) is accentuated. This, in turn, leads to a 'layering' of stigma over other forms of social inequalities, notably, gender, same-sex unions, transgender, drug use and mental and/or physical disability. It is argued by Porter (2014) that pointing the finger at less powerful groups helps non-marginalised groups feel less vulnerable and less at risk and gives a false sense of security as AIDS is seen as someone else's business. It is a case of moral prejudice driving the HIV epidemic (Porter 2014). Simbayi (2010) has said that entwined with reproducing structures of power structures, the social control model has helped explain the dynamics of stigma as related to complex social processes that act to reinforce existing social inequalities. Using the experience in the informal settlements of South Africa, xenophobia is highlighted as causing violence and conflict directed at outsiders held as responsible for the presence of HIV in their community. In these informal settlements, there is a tendency to blame a whole range of problems on foreigners that serves to further fuel a complex system of community xenophobia (Simbayi 2010).

Migrants, and in particular urban refugees, in the face of xenophobia, have traversed national borders and are widely documented as facing cultural and language barriers that hamper access to formal health care (IOM and APHRC 2015). This sense of marginalisation leaves the new urban arrival especially vulnerable particularly when seeking safety in the least regulated part of the city – the slum. The overall effect is of further marginalising minorities from accessing health care, which already exists sparingly in these deprived environments (IOM and APHRC 2015). Research by Porter (2014) has shown that marginalised mobile groups have often been displaced by violent conflict which includes migrants, refugees and internally displaced persons. Porter (2014) makes the point that these mobile groups are especially vulnerable to HIV in that they fall outside of the law, such as it exists in the slum environment. These groups can include undocumented migrants, internally displaced people as well as various rebel groups and ad hoc militia.

Rooted in global gender and economic inequalities, stigma relating to HIV is more intense for women than men (ICRW 2015). Often blamed for transmitting HIV, women living with HIV are often considered sexually promiscuous; conversely, men living with HIV are likely to be culturally absolved of blame for HIV infection and even applauded for remaining strong in the face of adversity (ICRW 2015). Deaths due to AIDS-related illness have led to further scapegoating and re-stigmatising of women blamed for their partner's HIV-related death (Munang'andu 2013). How this blaming is accepted or rejected and referenced against a given value system remains something of an unknown as well as the impact of socially ascribed shame through being held responsible for the spread of HIV. The adverse effect of shame, however, is widely covered elsewhere including in the context of poverty and humiliation (Zavaleta 2007).

Education, Health Care and Resilience

Life choices are greatly enhanced through education, if only through to secondary level (United Nations Educational, Scientific and Cultural Organization (UNESCO) 2014). Adolescents are more likely to have poor health status as adults if they have had little or no formal education in their formative years (Lloyd et al. 2004). A number of studies point to the direct connection between cumulative years of formal education and age of sexual initiation (Fatusi 2004; Okonkwo et al. 2005). Despite the 2003 launch of free primary education in Kenya, which led to an increase in uptake of formal education from 5.9 million in 2002 to 9.9 million in 2011, the quality of education has significantly declined in many government schools (Ngware et al. 2013). Numerous challenges to accessing formal education exist in the urban slum and in particular those to do with inadequate infrastructure and social amenities, makeshift classrooms, suboptimal construction standards and maintenance and absence of schools serving marginalised populations (UNESCO 2005; Government of Kenya 2005). In general, the shortage of government primary schools in slum settings and the high number – 80 per cent – of low-cost (private) schools not registered with the Ministry of Education deny many of the urban poor the opportunity of free primary education and the positive impact associated with formal education on health and livelihoods (Lloyd et al. 2004; Ngware et al. 2013).

In Nairobi, an increase of young people attaining secondary and tertiary levels of education between 2000 and 2012 is reported, a sign of a functioning 'urban advantage' (APHRC 2014). However this aggregate masks the substantial intra-urban differences between slum and non-slum areas. In the non-slum areas of the city, the proportion of young males to reach secondary or higher levels of education is 70.1 per cent compared with 52 per cent in the slums (APHRC 2014).

The literature points to a firm desire for education among slum-dwellers even if this means attending fee-paying private schools (UNESCO 2012). It is arguably an indication of community strength, of a steadfast resilience, as when schools close or when fees become unavailable, much effort is afforded by many slum residents to find the required resources to facilitate attendance in formal education (APHRC 2014). Education provides the resilience among slum-dwellers to effect meaningful change, or at least challenge the daily reality of life in the urban slum.

Whereas the data requires further disaggregation, research shows that schools are not always safe spaces for young people. Repeated abuse of adolescent girls by adult male teachers has been documented (Ngware et al. 2013). As Le Mat shows (2013), the reasons for this abuse have been cited as a demoralised teacher workforce in which employment in a run-down slum school is regarded as a 'dead end option'. It also demonstrates a lack of accountability for teachers' behaviour. The result is a deep distrust of formal institutions and, for many, a lasting fear of gender-based violence (Le Mat 2013). Within this climate of fear and distrust, children grow and mature into adults and with a world view shaped by prior experience. Explanations as to how young people perceive the origins of their vulnerability and identify the means of resilience remain a gap in the evidence and nowhere more so than in the study of HIV, dignity and reproductive health.

Explaining Vulnerability and Resilience: Modelling Health and Behaviour

Eaton et al. (2003) provide a cogent means of looking at HIV vulnerability drawing on social theory and backed by empirical evidence. For Eaton et al. (2003), the dynamics of HIV infection is observable on three interrelated levels: first, personal factors; second, the proximal context (interpersonal relationships and physical and organisational environment); and third, the distal context (culture and structural factors).

The literature demonstrates that the focus on personal factors, or individual agency, the 'behavioural approach', has continued to exert influence on western theories of risk and resilience (Smith 2003). Within this approach, adoption of risk reduction strategies is largely driven by subjective perception of one's own risk of infection. The behavioural approach recognises a strong correlation between knowledge and self-protection (Kohler et al. 2007; Smith 2003; King 1999). Vulnerability and ill health are evaluated against perceived health outcomes, forms of costs versus benefits analysis, perceived emotional and social consequences of potentially harmful behaviours and pressure to comply with shared interpretation of social norms (Eaton et al. 2003). Understanding personal factors, therefore, is the key to determining risky sexual behaviour and is at the heart of Social Cognitive Learning Theory influenced by behavioural and social psychology perspectives (Bandura 1991; Smith 2003). These perspectives underpin the Health Belief Model (Janz and Becker 1984; Rosenstock et al. 1994). Over the past 30 years, the Health Belief Model has been adapted to explain a variety of health behaviours, including sexual risk taking and the transmission of HIV. It is held that through a culturally sensitive study of personal attitudes and beliefs, accurate explanations and predictions can be constructed regarding key factors relating to the varying degrees of risk and resilience (Bandura 1991; Rosenstock et al. 1994).

Research carried out by Kibombo et al. (2007) in sub-Saharan Africa has examined the notion of 'correct assessment' of risk and resilience in the context of HIV among young people and has shown that personal assessment of a given situation is just as likely to be correct as it is to be incorrect. Mberu (2010) demonstrated that individual perception of risk has a direct bearing on adolescent health outcomes including unwanted pregnancy, unsafe abortion as well as drug and substance abuse. A body of evidence is emerging that demonstrates a degree of discordance between young people's sexual behaviour and individual risk perception. Simply being young, for many adolescents, and especially so for males, is considered as being resilient enough against HIV infection (Mberu 2010). This has led to questioning the process of knowledge translation at both an individual and collective level. Much of the discourse has looked at the notion of 'inaccurate perception' of risk coupled with the high levels of HIV among young people in urban slums and adolescent sexuality (Dann 2009; Ministry of Health, Uganda and ORC Macro 2006). In the study of risk perception towards sexually transmitted infections among young people, a twofold approach has been proposed which considers objective assessment that acknowledges a degree of risk of contracting HIV and the

'problematic discordant model', stemming from irrational decision-making including denial and rejection (Mberu 2010). The almost totally unexplored question of
sex addiction as a driving force for irrational risky behaviour is striking throughout
all models of health.

Shortcomings of the behavioural perspectives have been pointed out on different
levels (Mberu 2010). It is held that individual cognition models invariably favour
the 'western experience' and fail to appreciate the broader environmental and economic forces including the nature of 'protective sexual behaviour'. Empirical gaps
in evidence are apparent in the Health Belief Model which essentially emphasises
individual agency as the key unit of analysis when studying the subject of risky sex
while failing to account for structural determinants and lack of individual choice.
Moreover, in stressing personal responsibility, commentators have pointed to the
'blaming of the victim' as people may feel a sense of guilt for not solving their own
health problems even though the answer may lie in broader economic and/or environmental factors over which an individual has little control (Resource Centre for
Adolescent Pregnancy Prevention 2015). This has been documented elsewhere
(Lindner 2009) regarding the generation of a sense of humiliation for not dealing
with a potentially shaming event.

Vulnerability and risk are multifaceted concepts and do not fit easily into one
mode of enquiry or the confines of one theoretical position. In many instances, they
often co-exist as constructs and not as polar opposites. For Brockerhoff and
Biddlecom (1999), prior experiences and influence of current surroundings help
create perceptions of risk based on an interpretation of the severity of behavioural
outcomes, for example, acquiring HIV through risky sex. The influence of social
and cultural norms as well as peer interpretation are critical determinants of behaviour perceived as being either at high or low risk. For young people in particular, the
social environment plays a crucial role in health-related behaviour including friends
and peers, sexual partners, family members and immediate community (Okonkwo
et al. 2005). This has been demonstrated, for example, in regard to the impact of
young people's peer groups on their reproductive and sexual behaviour (Diclemente
1991; Stanton-Salazar and Urso Spina 2005). Stanton-Salazar and Urso Spina
(2005) have shown that health seeking is strongly influenced by the behaviour and
attitude of peers. For example, concerning the use of condoms, young people who
believe their peers are using condoms will more likely use condoms (Diclemente
1991, 1992; Stanton-Salazar and Urso Spina 2005).

Empirical literature repeatedly demonstrates that in understanding sexual risk
and behaviour, the discussion must go beyond that of individual subjective characteristics and focus more on objective proximal and distal factors (Eaton et al. 2003).
This approach sees cultural factors and dominant cultural and subcultural traditions
as forming the basis of analytical work on vulnerability and risk. Furthermore, the
study of structural factors including the legal, political, economic and organisational
environment is paramount (Eaton et al. 2003).

In studying the vulnerability of key populations, 'social behaviour' models take
as the point of departure, an analysis of the milieu of social influences that impact
on personal perception (King 1999). These models highlight social pressures, peer

influences, cultural expectations, economic factors, legal and political structures and political and religious systems which together present the individual with the range of options available and the means of disseminating information (Smith 2003). Social behaviour models have been viewed against 'rationalistic theories' of human behaviour highlighting the role of individual vulnerability as much as individual empowerment and resilience (Toroitich-Ruto 2001).

Attempts have been made to combine social learning theory and the structural-environmental models which together form the key theoretical perspectives for a contextual understanding of young people's reproductive and sexual behaviour (King 1999). Behaviour, risk and sexuality within structural-environmental theory since the early 1980s, has increasingly pointed to the function of individual, social, structural and environmental factors that provide a framework for seeing and studying the major factors relevant to adolescent reproductive behaviour and vulnerability (McLeroy et al. 1988; Sweat and Denison 1995).

Further insight into the importance of health and location has been offered by social epidemiology,[16] a relatively new and arguably contested branch of epidemiology (Jorgenson and Rice 2012). Jorgenson and Rice (2012), citing Berkman and Kawachi (2000) and Krieger (2001), state that in social epidemiological enquiry, the basic unit for analysis is the 'social-organisational production of disproportionate illness among disadvantaged segments of a population' (p. 103). This perspective is gradually moving away from a largely individual-level unit of analysis to a population-level perspective which seeks to understand large-scale structural arrangements and the socio-organisational patterns that influence health outcomes of a given population (Jorgenson and Rice 2012). Social epidemiology, inter alia, looks at levels of poverty, patterns of discrimination and the forms of inequality within a society that have a direct bearing on differential morbidity and mortality rates (Krieger 1999).

Contextual social determinants and their influence on health, wellbeing and risk have been described as constituting 'biological reflections of social fault lines' (Jorgenson and Rice 2012, p. 104), in which disease distribution follows patterns of power, privilege and inequality (Krieger 2001). In this light, urban slum prevalence is a dimension of the social production of morbidity and mortality stemming from prevailing social inequities and economic organisation that wholly characterise the urban slum.

As Jorgenson and Rice (2012), citing Engels (1845 (1968)) and Yankauer (1950), point out, demonstrating that social factors are key in shaping health and illness is nothing new. Social epidemiology, however, challenges the 'biomedical and de-socialised' model which focuses on individual-level biological and behavioural risk factors (Jorgenson and Rice 2012 citing: Berkman and Kawachi 2000; Farmer et al. 2006). The biomedical model emphasises the patterns of disease, whereas social epidemiology focuses more on the dynamics shaping susceptibility to ill health (Krieger 2001). Social epidemiological enquiry has been conceptualised as an examination of the totality of 'structural violence' (Farmer et al. 2006). Structural

---

[16] Social epidemiology has also been termed 'medical sociology'.

violence, in this sense, refers to the inequitable social order that disadvantages particular (marginalised) groups in society (Jorgenson and Rice 2012) and is manifested in individual-level pathology and population-level disparities in sickness and disease (Farmer 2000).

Behavioural economics has provided an analytical frame work and especially in regard to the interplay of objective characteristics and subjective experience (Samson 2014). A core theme is that perception of, and reaction to, reality is wholly subjective. How a young adolescent, for example, 'feels' about life is likely to be more important than an evaluation based solely on objective characteristics (Kahneman and Krueger 2006; Samson 2014). Samson (2014) explains how research on 'coherent arbitrariness' shows that people often have little idea about how to value a particular life experience. In another line of research, the rule of 'adaptation' has demonstrated the divide between objective characteristics of an experience and people's hedonic reactions to it and that through the process of 'hedonic adaptation' an individual adapts to diverse even contradictory experiences (Lyubomirsky 2012). In these perspectives, all judgement is relative (Samson 2014). This position finds is further expressed in 'prospect theory' which holds that all judgments of value are subjective and, therefore, relative (Kahneman and Tversky 1979). In short, perceptions matter more than reality. Furthermore, 'dual-system theory' especially as applied in cognitive and social psychology has explained why judgments and decisions often do not conform to formal notions of rationality (Frankish 2010). That is, the first system primarily concerns thinking processes that are largely experience based as well as relatively unconscious and the second system which is characterised as being controlled and deliberative (Samson 2014).

References

African Population and Health Research Center. (2002). *Nairobi informal settlements needs assessment survey.* Retrieved from http://www.chs.ubc.ca/archives/files/Health%20and%20 Livelihood%20Needs%20of%20Residents%20of%20Informal%20Settlements%20in%20 Nairobi%20City.pdf

African Population and Health Research Center. (2014). *Population and health dynamics in Nairobi's informal settlements. Report of the Nairobi Cross-sectional Slums Survey (NCSS) 2012.* Nairobi: African Population and Health Research Center.

African Union. (2013a, July 12–16). *Declaration of the special summit of the African Union on HIV/AIDS, tuberculosis and malaria: Abuja, Nigeria.* Retrieved from http://www.au.int/en/content/special-summit-african-union-hivaids-tuberculosis-and-malaria-abuja-nigeria

African Union. (2013b, December 30). *Second desk review/popular version: Women and girls, HIV/AIDS and conflicts: Situation analysis of 11 selected conflict and post- conflict countries in Africa.* Retrieved from http://www.aidswatchafrica.org/sites/default/files/publication-documents/2nd%20Desk%20Review%20Popular%20Report%20final%20copy.pdf

AIDSinfo. (2014). *Limitation to treatment safety and efficacy: Guidelines for the use of antiretrovial agents in HIV-1-infected adults and adolescents.* Retrieved from http://aidsinfo.nih.gov/guidelines/html/1/adult-and-adolescent-arv-guidelines/30/adherence-to-art

Amnesty International. (2009). *The unseen majority: Nairobi's two million slum-dwellers.* Retrieved from http://www.amnesty.org/en/documents/AFR32/005/2009/en/

Anderson, N., Cockcroft, A., & Shea, B. (2008). Gender-based violence and HIV: Relevance for HIV prevention in hyperendemic countries of southern Africa. *AIDS, 22*(Suppl 4), 73–86. doi:10.1097/01.aids.0000341778.73038.86.

Bandura, A. (1991). A social cognitive approach to the exercise of control over AIDS infection. In R. Diclemente (Ed.), *Adolescent and AIDS: A generation in jeopardy* (pp. 25–59). New York: Plenum.

Barbieri, M., & Hertrich, V. (2005). Age difference between spouses and contraceptive practice in sub-Saharan Africa. *Population, 60*(5/6), 617–654. Retrieved from http://search.proquest.com/docview/196905383?pq-origsite=gscholar

Basic Education Coalition. (2015). *Overview of millennium development goals.* Retrieved from Basic Education Coalition website: http://www.basiced.org/basic/overview-of-millenium-development-goals/

Berkman, L. F., & Kawachi, I. (Eds.). (2000). *A historical framework for social epidemiology.* New York: Oxford University Press.

Brake, M. (2013). *The sociology of youth culture and youth subcultures: Sex and drugs and rock 'n' roll?* Routledge Revivals.

Brockerhoff, M., & Biddlecom, A. E. (1999). Migration, sexual behaviour and the risk of HIV in Kenya. *International Migration Review, 33*(4), 833–856.

Browing, R. B., Leventhal, T., & Brooks-Gunn, J. (2005). Sexual initiation in early adolescence: The nexus of parental and community control. *American Sociological Review, 70*(5), 758–778. Retrieved from http://asr.sagepub.com/content/70/5/758.abstract

Burns, P. A., & Snow, R. C. (2012). The built environment & the impact of neighborhood characteristics on youth sexual risk behavior in Cape Town, South Africa. *Health & Place, 18*(5), 1088–1100. doi:10.1016/j.healthplace.2012.04.013.

Caldwell, B. (2014). Why mothers in slums may prefer the informal health care sector: Lessons from Dhaka Bangladesh. *OpenPop.* Retrieved from http://www.openpop.org/?p=889

Chambers, R. (1995). Poverty and livelihoods: whose reality counts? *Environment and Urbanization, 7*(1), 173–202. Retrieved from http://eau.sagepub.com/content/7/1/173.full.pdf

Chant, S. (1997). *Women-headed households. Diversity and dynamics in the developing world.* Basingstoke: Macmillan Press.

Cleary, S. M., Birch, S., Moshabela, M., & Schneider, H. (2012). Unequal access to ART: Exploratory results from rural and urban case studies of ART use. *Sexually Transmitted Infection, 88*(2), 141–146. doi:10.1136/sextrans-2011-050136.

Collazzoni, A., Capanna, C., Bustini, M., Stratta, P., Ragusa, M., Marino, A., & Rossi, A. (2014). Research report humiliation and interpersonal sensitivity in depression. *Journal of Affective Disorders, 167*, 224–227. doi:10.1016/j.jad.2014.06.008.

Cotton, C. (2013). *Research to practice – Strengthening contributions to evidence-based policy making.* Retrieved from https://www.mcqil.ca/isid/files/isid/pd2013cotton.pdf

Dann, G. (2009). Sexual behaviour and contraceptive use among youth in West Africa 2001. *Population Reference Bureau, Publications.* Retrieved from http://www.prb.org/Publications/Articles/2009/westafricayouth.aspx

David, A. M., Mercado, S. P., Becker, D., Edmundo, K., & Mugisha, F. (2007). The prevention and control of HIV/AIDS, TB and Vector-borne diseases in informal settlements: Challenges, opportunities and insights. *Journal of Urban Health, 84*(1), 65–74. Retrieved from http://www.ncbi.nlm.nih.gov/pubmed/17431796

Dick, B. (2013). *Strengthening national responses to HIV and adolescents in emergency situations, lessons learned from Cote d'Ivoire and Haiti.* New York: UNICEF.

DiClemente, R. J. (1991). Predictors of HIV-preventive sexual behaviour in a high-risk adolescent population: The influence of perceived peer norms and sexual communication on incarcerated adolescents' consistent use of condoms. *Journal of Adolescents Health, 12*(5), 385–390. Retrieved from http://www.ncbi.nlm.nih.gov/pubmed/1751507

DiClemente, R. J. (1992). Psychological determinants of condom use among adolescents. In R. J. DiClemente (Ed.), *Adolescents and AIDS: A generation in jeopardy* (pp. 34–51). Thousand Oaks: Sage Publications.

Dobransky, P. (2015). Sex as a social currency. *Self-growth.com*. Retrieved from http://www.self-growth.com/articles/sex-as-a-social-currency

Dodoo, F. N.-A., Zulu, E. M., & Ezeh, A. C. (2007). Urban–rural differences in the socioeconomic deprivation–Sexual behaviour link in Kenya. *Social Science & Medicine, 64*(5), 1019–1031. doi:10.1016/j.socscimed.2006.10.007.

Dugan, L. (2011, December 16). Safe and secure housing is critical to the wellbeing of mental health patients. *Health Service Journal*. Retrieved from http://www.hsj.co.uk/comment/blogs/leadership-in-mental-health/safe-and-secure-housing-is-critical-to-the-wellbeing-of-mental-health-patients/5039455.blog

Durand-Lasserve, A., & Selod, H. (2009). The formalization of urban land tenure in developing countries. In S. V. Lall, M. Friere, B. Yuen, R. Rajack, & J. J. Helluin (Eds.), *Urban land markets – Improving land management for successful urbanization* (pp. 101–132). Netherlands: Springer. doi:10.1007/978-1-4020-8862-9.

Eaton, L., Flisher, A. J., & Aarø, L. E. (2003). Unsafe sexual behaviour in South African youth. *Social Science and Medicine, 56*(1), 149–165. doi:10.1016/S0277-9536(02)00017-5.

Egondi, T., Kyobutungi, C. N., Muindi, K., Oti, S., Van de Viger, S., Ettarh, R., & Rocklov, J. (2013). Communication perceptions of air pollution and related health risks in Nairobi in slums. *International Journal of Environmental Research and Public Health, 10*(10), 4851–4868. doi:10.3390/ijerph10104851.

Ekdale, B. (2011). *A history of Kibera*. Retrieved from http://www.brianekdale.com/uploads/kiberahistory.pdf

Engels, F. (1845 [1968]). *The condition of the working class in England*. Stanford: Stanford University Press.

Farmer, P. E. (2000). Infections and inequalities: The modern plagues. *Medical Anthropology Quarterly, New Series, 14*(3), 448. Retrieved from http://www.jstor.org/stable/i226521

Farmer, P. E., Nizeye, B., Stulac, S., & Keshavjee, S. (2006). Structural violence and clinical medicine. *PLoS Medicine, 3*(10), 1686–1691. doi:10.1371/journal.pmed.0030449.

Fatusi, A. O. (2004). *Study of African universities response to HIV/AIDS* (Report submitted to the Association of the Africa University, Ghana). Ibadan: The Nigerian Universities.

Fineman, N. (2008). The social construction of noncompliance: A study of health care and social service providers in everyday practice. *Sociology of Health & Illness, 13*(3), 354–374. doi:10.1111/1467-9566.ep10492252.

Fotso, J. C., Ezeh, A., & Oronje, R. (2008). Provision and use of maternal health services among urban poor women in Kenya: What do we know and what we can we do? *Journal of Urban Health, 85*(3), 428–442. doi:10.1007/s11524-008-9263-1.

Fotso, J. C., Ezeh, A., Madise, N., Ziraba, A., & Ogollah, R. (2009). What does access to maternal care mean among the urban poor? Factors associated with use of appropriate maternal health services in the slum settlements of Nairobi, Kenya. *Maternal Child Health Journal, 13*(1), 130–137. doi:10.1007/s10995-008-0326-4.

Frankish, K. (2010). Dual-process and dual-system theories of reasoning. *Philosophy Compass, 5*(10), 914–992. doi:10.1111/j.1747-9991.2010.00330.x.

Fustos, K. (2011). *Gender-based violence increases risk of HIV/AIDS for women in sub-Saharan Africa*. Population Reference Bureau Publications. Retrieved from http://www.prb.org/Publications/Articles/2011/gender-based-violence-hiv.aspx

Garenne, M. (2010). Urbanization and child health in resource poor settings with special reference to under five mortality in Africa. *Archives of Diseases in Childhood, 95*(6), 464–468. doi:10.1136/adc.2009.172585.

Glaeser, E. L., Kahn, M. E., & Rappaport, J. (2008). Why do the poor live in cities? The role of public transportation. *Journal of Urban Economics, 63*(1), 1–24. doi:10.1016/j.jue.2006.12.004.

Goodman, G. S., & Hilton, A. A. (2010). Urban dropouts: Why persist? (chap. 4). *Counterpoints, 215*(19). In *Urban questions: Teaching in the city: second edition* (pp. 55–67). Peter Lang AG.

Government of Kenya. (2005). *Meeting the challenges of education training and research in Kenya in the 21st century. A policy framework for education, training and research* (Sessional Paper No 1). Nairobi: Government of Kenya.

Greif, M. J. (2012). Housing, medical, and food deprivation in poor urban contexts: Implications for multiple sexual partnerships and transactional sex in Nairobi's slums. *Health & Place, 18*(2), 400–407. doi:10.1016/j.healthplace.2011.12.008.

Hartling, L., Lindner, E., Spalthoff, U., & Britton, M. (2013). Humiliation: A nuclear bomb of emotions? *Psicología Política, 46*, 55–76. Retrieved from http://www.uv.es/garzon/psicologia%20politica/N46-3.pdf

Heflin, C. M., & Iceland, J. (2009). Poverty, material hardship, and depression. *Social Science Quarterly, 90*(5), 1051–1071. Retrieved from http://onlinelibrary.wiley.com/doi/10.1111/j.1540-6237.2009.00645.x/pdf

Home Grown School Feeding. (2015). *Orphans and vulnerable children defined.* Retrieved from Home Grown School Feeding website: http://hgsf-global.org/en/ovc/background/263-orphans-andvulnerable-children-defined

Human Rights Watch. (2010). *Protect health workers, activists, condemn mob violence, incitements to hate. (Halt anti-gay campaign). Human rights watch.* Retrieved from http://www.hrw.org/news/2010/02/17/kenya-halt-anti-gay-campaign

International Centre for Research on Women. (2015). *Stigma and discrimination.* Retrieved from http://www.icrw.org/what-we-do/hiv-aids/stigma-discrimination

International Organization for Migration (IOM). (2011a). *Integrated biological and behavioural surveillance survey among migrant female sex workers in Nairobi, Kenya 2010. Healthy migrants in healthy communities.* Retrieved from the International Organization for Migration website: http://health.iom.int/

International Organization for Migration (IOM). (2011b). *An analysis of migration health in Kenya – Healthy migrants in healthy communities.* Retrieved from the International Organization for Migration website: http://health.iom.int/

International Organization for Migration (IOM). (2011c). *IOM, glossary on migration* (International Migration Law Series No. 25). Retrieved from https://www.iom.int/key-migration-terms.

IOM and APHRC (2015). Regional synthesis on patterns and determinants of migrants' health and associated vulnerabilities in urban setting of East and Southern Africa. Johannesburg: International Organization on Migration.

Isunju, J. B., Schwartz, K., Schouten, M. A., Johnson, W. P., & van Diik, M. M. (2011). Socio-economic aspects of improved sanitation in slums: A review. *Public Health, 125*(6), 368–376. doi:10.1016/j.puhe.2011.03.008.

Izugbara, C. O., & Ngilangwa, D. P. (2010). Women, poverty and adverse maternal outcomes in Nairobi, Kenya. *BioMed Centre, Women's Health, 10*(33), 2–8. doi:10.1186/1472-6874-10-33.

Jaftha, T. (2015, May 12). Xenophobia' in South Africa: Order, chaos, and the moral degradation of the rainbow nation. *Bonfiire Stellenbosch.* Retrieved from http://www.bonfiire.com/stellenbosch/2015/05/xenophobia-in-south-africa-order-chaos-and-the-moral-degradation-of-the-rainbow-nation/

Janz, N. K., & Becker, M. H. (1984). The health belief model: A decade later. *Health Education Quarterly, 11*(1), 1–47. doi:10.1177/109019818401100101.

Jasinski, J. L., Wesely, J. K., Mustaine, E., & Wright, J. D. (2005). *The experience of violence in the lives of homeless women: a research report.* Retrieved from http://www.ncjrs.gov/pdffiles1/nij/grants/211976.pdf

Joint United Nations Programme on HIV/AIDS (UNAIDS). (2011a). *Place matters HIV in the city.* Unpublished raw data.

Joint United Nations Programme on HIV/AIDS (UNAIDS). (2011b). *A new investment framework for the global HIV response* (UNAIDS Issues Brief). Geneva: UNAIDS.

Joint United Nations Programme on HIV/AIDS (UNAIDS). (2013a). *Global AIDS progress report.* Kenya. Retrieved from www.unaids.org/AIDSReporting

Joint United Nations Programme on HIV/AIDS (UNAIDS). (2013b). *Global epidemic.* Geneva: UNAIDS.

Joint United Nations Programme on HIV/AIDS (UNAIDS). (2013c). *Towards strategic investments in HIV and AIDS at city level: Lessons learnt from the known epidemic response exercise in Windhoek, Namibia.* Geneva: UNAIDS.

Joint United Nations Programme on HIV/AIDS (UNAIDS). (2014a). *UNAIDS briefing book July 2014*. Geneva: UNAIDS.

Joint United Nations Programme on HIV/AIDS (UNAIDS). (2014b). *The gap report*. Geneva: UNAIDS.

Joint United Nations Programme on HIV/AIDS (UNAIDS). (2014c). *The cities report*. Retrieved from http://issuu.com/pm.dstaids.sp/docs/jc2687_thecitiesreport_en

Jorgenson, A. K., & Rice, J. (2012). Urban slums and children's health. In F. A. Karides (Ed.) *Journal of World-Systems Research, 18*(1), 103–116. Retrieved from http://www.jwsr.org/wp-content/uploads/2013/02/jorgensonrice-vol18n1.pdf

Kabiru, C. W. (2015, June 16). Are we failing adolescent girls? *APHRC*. Retrieved from http://aphrc.org/are-we-failing-adolescent-girls/

Kahneman, D. K., & Krueger, A. B. (2006). Developments in the measurements of subjective well-being. *The Journal of Economic Perspectives, 20*(1), 3–24. doi:10.1257/089533006776526030.

Kahneman, D. K., & Tversky, A. (1979). Prospect theory: An analysis of decision under risk. *Econometrica, 47*(2), 263. doi:10.2307/1914185.

Kamndaya, M., Thomas, L., Vearey, J., Sartorius, B., & Kazembe, L. (2014). Material deprivation affects high sexual risk behavior among young people in urban slums, South Africa. *Journal of Urban Health, 91*(3), 581–591. doi:10.1007/s11524-013-9856-1.

Kamungi, P. (2013). *Municipalities and IDPs outside of camps: The case of Kenya's 'integrated' displaced persons*. Retrieved from http://reliefweb.int/report/kenya/municipalities-and-idps-outside-camps-case-kenya%E2%80%99s-%E2%80%98integrated%E2%80%99-displaced-persons

Kenya Human Rights Commission & Reproductive Health and Rights Alliance. (2010). *Teenage pregnancy and unsafe abortion; the case of Korogocho slums*. Retrieved from http://hdl.handle.net/123456789/84

Khan, M. M. H., Grübner, O., & Krämer, A. (2012). Frequently used healthcare services in urban slums of Dhaka and adjacent rural areas and their determinants. *Journal of Public Health, 34*(2), 261–271. doi:10.1093/pubmed/fdr108.

Kibombo, R., Neema, S., & Ahmed, F. H. (2007). Perceptions of risk to HIV infection among adolescents in Uganda: Are they related to sexual behaviour? *African Journal of Reproductive Health, 11*(3), 168–181. Retrieved from http://www.ncbi.nlm.nih.gov/pubmed/18458740

King, R. (1999). *Sexual behavior change for HIV: Where have theories taken us?* (Key Material No. UNAIDS/99.27E). Retrieved from http://www.popline.org/node/533607#sthash.KICxIgul.dpuf

Kjellstrom, T., Friel, S., Dixon, J., Corvalan, C., Rehfuess, E., Campbell-Lendrum, D., Gore, F., & Bartram, J. (2007). Urban environmental health hazards and health equity. *Journal of Urban Health, 84*(1), 86–97. doi:10.1007/s11524-007-9171-9.

Kohler, H. P., Behrman, J. R., & Watkins, S. C. (2007). Social networks and HIV/AIDS risk perceptions. *Demography, 44*(1), 1–33. doi:10.1353/dem.2007.0006.

Krieger, N. (1999). Embodying inequality: A review of concepts, measures, and methods for studying health consequences of discrimination. *International Journal of Health Services, 29*(2), 295–352. doi:http://dx.doi.org/10.2190/M11W-VWXE-KQM9-G97Q.

Krieger, N. (2001). Theories for social epidemiology in the 21st century: An ecosocial perspective. *International Journal of Epidemiology, 30*(4), 668–677. doi:10.1093/ije/30.4.668.

Kushel, M. B., Gupta, R., Gee, L., & Haas, J. S. (2006). Housing instability and food insecurity as barriers to healthcare among low-income Americans. *Journal of General Internal Medicine, 21*(1), 71–77. doi:10.1111/j.1525-1497.2005.00278.x.

Kyobutungi, C., Ziraba, A. K., Ezeh, A., & Yé, Y. (2008). *The burden of disease profile of residents of Nairobi's slums: Results from a demographic surveillance*. doi:10.1186/1478-7954-6-1.

Le Mat, M. (2013). *Perspectives from teachers and students in a secondary school in Addis Ababa, Ethiopia*. Retrieved from http://www.africabib.org/rec.php?RID=Q00030803&DB=p

Lederer, E. M. (2011, March 25). 27.5 million internally displaced by violence. *The Associated Press*. Retrieved from http://www.bing.com/videos/search?q=27.5+million+internally+displaced+by+violence&qpvt=27.5+Million+internally+displaced+by+violence&FORM=VDRE

Leidner, B., Sheikh, H., & Ginges, J. (2012). Affective dimensions of intergroup humiliation. *PLoS One*. doi:10.1371/journal.pone.0046375.

Lindner, E. (2001). Humiliation and the human condition: Mapping a minefield. *Human Rights Review, 2*(2), 46–63. Retrieved from http://www.humiliationstudies.org/documents/evelin/MappingMinefield.pdf

Lindner, E. (2006). *Making enemies. Humiliation and international conflict.* Westport/London: Greenwood/Praeger Security International.

Lindner, E. (2009). *Emotion and conflict: How human rights can dignify emotion and help us wage good conflict.* Westport/London: Praeger.

Lindner, E. (2010). *Gender, humiliation and global security, dignifying relationships from love, sex, and parenthood to world affairs.* Santa Barbara: Prager Security International.

Lindner, E. (2012). *A dignity economy: Creating an economy that serves human dignity and preserves our planet.* Oslo: Dignity Press.

Lloyd, D., Newall, S., & Dietrick, E. C. (2004). *Health inequity: A review of the literature.* Retrieved from ePublications@SCU.

Luke, N. (2005). Confronting the 'sugar daddy' stereotype: Age and economic asymmetries and risky sexual behavior in urban Kenya. *International Family Planning Perspectives, 31*(1), 6–14. Retrieved from http://www.jstor.org/stable/3649496

Luke, N., Xu, H., Mberu, B. U., & Goldberg, R. E. (2012). Migration experience and premarital sexual initiation in urban Kenya: An event history analysis. *Studies in Family Planning, 43*(2), 115–126. Retrieved from http://www.ncbi.nlm.nih.gov/pmc/articles/PMC3665273/

Lyubomirsky, S. (2012). *The myths of happiness: What should make you happy, but doesn't, what shouldn't make you happy, but does.* London: Penguin Press.

Martin, D. C. (2008). Experience of homeless people in the health care delivery system: A descriptive phenomenological study. *Public Health Nurse, 25*(5), 420–430. doi:10.1111/j.1525-1446. 2008.00726.x.

Mberu, B. U. (2010). Risk perception for HIV/AIDS infection among premarital sexuality initiated youth in Nigeria. *African Population Studies, 24*(3), 188–210. doi:http://dx.doi.org/10.11564/24-3-299.

Mberu, B. U. (2012, November 11). *Adolescent sexual and reproductive health and rights: Research evidence from sub-Saharan Africa.* PPD conference "Evidence for action: South-south collaboration for ICPD beyond 2014," Ruposhi Bangla Hotel, Dhaka. Abstract retrieved from http://r4d.dfid.gov.uk/PDF/Outputs/StepUp/2012_PPDMberu.pdf

McCord, J. (1997). *Placing urban violence in context in violence and childhood in the inner city.* Cambridge: Cambridge University Press.

McLeroy, K. R., Bibeau, D., Steckler, A., & Glanz, K. (1988). An ecological perspective on health promotion programs. *Health Education Quarterly, 15*(4), 351–377. Retrieved from http://www.ncbi.nlm.nih.gov/pubmed/3068205

Metcalfe, V., Pavanello, S. with Mishra, P. (2011). *Sanctuary in the city? Urban displacement and vulnerability in Nairobi* (Overseas Development Institute, Humanitarian Policy Group Working Paper). London: Overseas Development Institute.

Miller, K. E., & Rasmussen, A. (2010). War exposure, daily stressors, and mental health in conflict and post-conflict settings: Bridging the divide between trauma-focused and psychosocial frameworks. *Social Science & Medicine, 70*(1), 7–16. doi:10.1016/j.socscimed. 2009.09.029.

Ministry of Health Uganda, & ORC Macro. (2006). *Uganda HIV/AIDS sero-behavioural survey 2004–2005.* Calverton: ORC Macro.

Moser, C. O. (2004). Urban violence and insecurity: An introductory roadmap. *Environment and Urbanization, 16*(2), 1–16. Retrieved from http://www.brookings.edu/research/opinions/2004/10/communitydevelopment-moser

Mumah, J., Kabriru, C. W., Izugbara, C., & Mukiira, C. (2014, April). *Coping with unintended pregnancies: Narratives from adolescents in Nairobi's slums* (Research Report). Retrieved from www.aphrc.org

Munang'andu, J. H. (2013, September 13). HIV/AIDS stigma and discrimination is worse than racism or cancer. *Modern Ghana*. Retrieved from http://www.modernghana.com/news/486789/1/hivaids-related-stigma-and-discrimination-is-worse.html

Mutisya, E. (2010). *The sustainability of downscaling of microfinance in Africa: Empirical evidence from Kenya*. Saarbrücken: VDM Verlag.

Mutisya, E., & Yarime, M. (2011). Understanding the grassroots dynamics of slums in Nairobi: The dilemma of Kibera informal settlements. *International Transactional Journal of Engineering, Management & Applied Sciences and Technologies, 2*(2), 197–212. Retrieved from http://TuEngr.com/V02/197-213.pdf

Ndugwa, R. P., Kabiru, C. W., Cleland, J., Beguy, D., Egondi, T., Zulu, E. M., & Jessor, R. (2011). Adolescent problem behavior in Nairobi's informal settlements: Applying problem behavior theory in sub-Saharan Africa. *Journal of Urban Health, 88*(2), 298–317. doi:10.1007/s11524-010-9462-4.

Ngware, M., Abuya, B., Admassu, K., Mutisya, M., Musyoka, P., & Oketch, M. (2013). *Quality and access to education in urban informal settlements in Kenya*. Retrieved from http://aphrc.org/publications/quality-and-access-to-education-in-urban-informal-settlements-in-kenya/

Oduro, G. Y., Swartz, S., & Arnot, M. (2012). Gender-based violence: Young women's experiences in the slums and streets of three sub-Saharan African cities. *Theory and Research in Education, 10*(3), 257–294. doi:10.1177/1477878512459395.

Okonkwo, P. I., Fatusi, A. O., & Ilika, A. L. (2005). Perceptions of peers' behaviour regarding sexual health decision making among female undergraduates in Anambra State, Nigeria. *African Health Science, 5*(2), 107–113. Retrieved from http://www.ncbi.nlm.nih.gov/pmc/articles/PMC1831917/

Okonofua, F. (2007). New research findings on adolescents reproductive health in Africa. *African Journal of Reproductive Health, 11*(3), 7–9.

Pamoja Trust. (2009). *An inventory of the slums in Nairobi*. Nairobi: Matrix Consultants.

Parks, M. (2014). Urban poverty traps: Neighbourhoods and violent victimisation and offending in Nairobi, Kenya. *Urban Studies, 51*(9), 1812–1832. doi:10.1177/0042098013504144.

Plummer, D. & McLean, A. (2010). The price of prejudice: The corrosive effect of HIV-related stigma on individuals and society (chap. 16). In M. Morrisssey, M. Bernd & D. Bundy (Eds.), *Challenging HIV and AIDS: A new role for Caribbean education* (pp. 232–239). Paris: United Nations Educational, Scientific and Cultural Organization.

Porter, A. (2014, March 14). Moral prejudice drives HIV/AIDS. *Cape Times*. Retrieved from http://www.ccr.org.za/index.php/media-release/in-the-media/newspaper-articles/item/1123-hiv-aids

Premji, S. N. (2014). Child care in crisis. *World Policy Journal, 31*(2), 81–89. doi:10.1177/0740277514541060.

Resource Centre for Adolescents Pregnancy Prevention (ReCAPP). (2015). *The health belief model*. Retrieved from ReCAPP website: http://recapp.etr.org/recapp/index.cfm?fuseaction+pages.TheoriesDetails&PageID=350

Rosenstock, I., Strecher, V., & Becker, M. (1994). The health belief model and HIV risk behaviour change. In R. J. DiClimente, & J. L. Peterson (Eds.), *Preventing AIDS: Theories and methods of behavioural interventions* (pp. 5–24). doi:10.1007/978-1-4899-1193-3_2.

Samson, A. (Ed.). (2014). *The behavioral economics guide 2014* (1st ed.). Retrieved from http://www.behavioraleconomics.com

Sclar, E. D., Garau, P., & Carolini, G. (2005). The 21st century health challenge of slums and cities. *The Lancet, 365*(9462), 901–903. Retrieved from http://ars.els-cdn.com/content/image/B01406736.gif

Scott-Storey, K., Wuest, J., & Ford-Gilboe, M. (2009). Intimate partner violence and cardiovascular risk: Is there a link? *Journal of Advanced Nursing, 65*(10), 2186–2197. doi:10.1111/j.1365-2648.2009.05086.x.

Sekudu, B. (2014). Mob justice on the rise in Ndofaya: Police against community's illegal actions. *Soweto Urban, Caxton Urban Newspapers*. Retrieved from http://www.bizcommunity.com/Article/196/90/6156.html

Shetty, P. (2011). Health care for the urban poor falls through the gap. *The Lancet, 377*(9766), 627–628. doi:http://dx.doi.org/10.1016/S0140-6736(11)60215-8.

Siegel, L., & El-Sadr, W. (2006). New perspectives in HIV treatment interruption: The SMART study. *Physicians Research Network.* Retrieved from http://www.prn.org/index.php/management/article/hiv_treatment_interruption

Simbayi, L. C. (2010, December 1). *The layering of HIV-related stigma within a community.* Presentation to the international conference on HIV-related stigma at Howard University. Abstract retrieved from http://whocanyou.s462.sureserver.com/wp-ontent/uploads/2011/02/LeicknessSimbayi.pdf

Smith, D. J. (2003). Imagining HIV/AIDS: Morality and perceptions of personal risk in Nigeria. *Journal of Medical Anthropology, 22*(4), 343–372. doi:10.1177/004208168702300206.

Springer, K. W., Sheridan, J., & Carnes, M. (2003). The long-term health outcomes of childhood abuse: An overview and a call to action. *Journal of General Internal Medicine, 18*(10), 864–870. doi:10.1046/j./1525-1497.2003.20918.x.

Stanton-Salazar, R. D., & Urso Spina, S. (2005). Adolescent peer networks as a context for social and emotional support. *Youth Society, 36*(4), 379–417. doi:10.1177/0044118X04267814.

Sweat, M., & Denison, J. (1995). Reducing HIV incidence in developing countries with structural and environmental interventions. *AIDS, 9*(Suppl A), 251–257. Retrieved from https://www.researchgate.net/publication/14384926_Sweat_M.D.__Denison_J.A._Reducing_HIV_incidence_in_developing_countries_with_structural_and_environmental_interventions._AIDS_9_S251-S257

Taffa, N., Chepngeno, G., & Amuyunzu-Nyamongo, M. (2005). Child morbidity and healthcare utilization in the slums of Nairobi, Kenya. *Journal of Tropical Pediatrics, 51*(5), 279–284. doi:10.1093/tropej/fmi012.

Tavory, I., & Swidler, A. (2009). Condom semiotics: Meaning and condom use in rural Malawi. *American Sociological Review, 74*(2), 171–189. doi:10.1177/000312240907400201.

Teruya, C., Longshore, D., Andersen, R. M., Arangua, L., Nyamathi, A., Leake, B., & Gelberg, L. (2010). Health and health care disparities among homeless women. *Women and Health, 50*(8), 719–736. doi:10.1080/03630242.2010.532754.

Centre on Housing Rights and Evictions (2005). Listening to the Poor: Housing Rights in Nairobi, Kenya. Consultation Report. Geneva: Centre on Housing Rights and Evictions

The American College of Obstetricians and Gynaecologists. (2013). *Health care for homeless women.* Committee on Health Care for Underserved Women. Retrieved from http://www.acog.org/Resources-And-Publications/committee-opinions/committee-on-health-care-for-underserved-women/Health-care-for-Homeless-women

The National Alliance to End Homelessness. (2012). *The state of homelessness in America.* Washington, DC: NAEH.

Thompson, C. (2011). *Neo-Marxist perspectives of crime.* Retrieved from https://sociologytwynham.wordpress.com

Toroitich-Ruto, C. (2001). The effect of HIV/AIDS on sexual behaviour of young people in Kenya. *African Population Studies, 12*(2), 39–50.

Turan, M. T., & Besirli, A. (2008). Impacts of the urbanisation process on mental health. *Anatolian Journal of Psychiatry, 9,* 238–243. Retrieved from https://www.researchgate.net/publication/36448313_Impacts_of_urbanization_process_on_ment

Unger, A., & Riley, L. W. (2007). Slum health: From understanding to action. *PLoS Medicine, 4*(10), 295. doi:10.1371/journal.pmed.0040295.

United Nations Children's Fund (UNICEF). (2012). *State of the world's children. Children in an urban world.* Retrieved from http://www.unicef.org/sowc2012/

United Nations Development Programme (UNDP). (2012a). *Global commission on HIV and the law. Risk, rights and health.* Retrieved from http://hivlawcommission.org/

United Nations Development Programme (UNDP). (2012b). *Lost in transition: Transgender people, rights and HIV vulnerability in the Asia-Pacific region.* Retrieved from http://www.undp.org/content/dam/undp/library/hivaids/UNDP_HIV_Transgender_report_Lost_in_Transition_May_2012.pdf

United Nations Educational, Scientific and Cultural Organization (UNESCO). (2005). *Challenges of implementing free primary education in Kenya. Assessment report.* Retrieved from http://unesdoc.unesco.org/images/0015/001516/151654eo.pdf

United Nations Educational, Scientific and Cultural Organization (UNESCO). (2012). *World Atlas of Gender Equality in Education* Paris: UNESCO

United Nations Educational, Scientific and Cultural Organization (UNESCO). (2014). *World Conference on Education for Sustainable Development.* Aichai-Nagoya, Japan, 10-12 November, 2014. Retrieved http://www.unesco.org/new/en/unesco-world-conference-on-esd-2014

United Nations Fund Population Fund (UNFPA). (2003). *Investment in adolescents' reproductive health is critical to fighting poverty and HIV/AIDS.* Retrieved from http://www.unfpa.org/news/investment-adolescents-reproductive-health-critical-fighting-poverty-and-hivaids-says-unfpa#sthash.9Qv4ixRo.dpuf

United Nations Fund Population Fund (UNFPA). (2008). *HIV interventions for young people in humanitarian emergencies. Global guidance briefs.* Retrieved from www.unfpa.org/hiv/iattdocs/humanitarian.pdf

United Nations Fund Population Fund (UNFPA). (2014). *Annual report.* Retrieved from http://www.unfpa.org/annual-report

United Nations Human Settlements Programme (UN-Habitat). (2003a). *Global report on human settlements: The challenge of slums.* Retrieved from http://mirror.unhabitat.org/pmss/listItemDetails.aspx?publicationID=1156

United Nations Human Settlements Programme (UN–Habitat). (2003b). *Slums of the world: The face of urban poverty in the new millennium?* (Working Paper). Retrieved from http://mirror.unhabitat.org/pmss/listItemDetails.aspx?publicationID=1124

United Nations Human Settlements Programme (UN–Habitat). (2007a). *Kenya slum upgrading project.* Strategy Document. Retrieved from http://nairobiplanninginnovations.com/projects/kenya-slum-upgrading-programme-kensup/

United Nations Human Settlements Programme (UN–Habitat). (2007b). *Enhancing urban safety and security. Global report on human settlements.* Retrieved from http://unhabitat.org/

United Nations Human Settlements Programme (UN–Habitat). (2010). *State of the world's cities 2010/2011. Cities for all: Bridging the urban divide.* Retrieved from http://unhabitat.org/

United Nations Human Settlements Programme (UN–Habitat). (2011). *23rd Governing Council of UN-Habitat.* Retrieved from http://unhabitat.org/

United Nations Human Settlements Programme (UN–Habitat). (2012). *Contribution of UN-Habitat to the annual MDG report.* Retrieved from http://unhabitat.org/

United Nations Human Settlements Programme (UN–Habitat). (2013a). *State of urban youth report 2012/2013. Youth in the prosperity of cities.* Retrieved from http://issuu.com/unhabitatyouthunit/docs/state_of_the_urban_yourh_report_201

United Nations Human Settlements Programme (UN–Habitat). (2013b). *Streets as public spaces and drivers of urban prosperity.* Retrieved from http://unhabitat.org/books/streets-as-public-spaces-and-drivers-of-urban-prosperity/

United Nations Office on Drugs and Crime (UNODC). (2012). *World drug report 2012.* Retrieved from http://www.unodc.org/unodc/en/data-and-analysis/WDR-2012.html

United Nations Population Division. (1998). *World population monitoring 1977.* Retrieved from http://www.un.org/esa/population/pubsarchive/catalogue/catrpt1.htm

Vijayaraghavan, M., Kushel, M. B., Vittinghoff, E., Kertesz, S., Jacobs, D., Lewis, C. E., Sidney, S., Bibbins-Domingo, K., & Cohort, M. (2013). Housing instability and incident hypertension in the Cardia cohort. *Journal of Medical Health, 90*(3), 427–441. Retrieved from doi:10.1007/s11524-012-9729-z.

Vivaldi Partners. (2010). *Social currency. Why brands need to build and nurture social currency.* Retrieved from http://images.fastcompany.com/Vivald-iPartners_Social-Currency.pdf

WebMd. (2014). High-risk sexual behavior. *Topic Overview Sexual Health Centre.* Retrieved from http://www.webmd.com/sex/tc/high-risk-sexual-behavior-topic-overview

Wikipedia. (2015). *Street children.* Retrieved from http://en.wikipedia.org/wiki/street_children

Wilkinson, R., & Marmot, M. (Eds.). (2003). *Social determinants of health, the solid facts* (2nd ed.). Copenhagen: World Health Organization/WHO Regional Office for Europe.

Williams, L. D. (2014). Understanding the relationships among HIV/AIDS-related stigma, health service utilization, and HIV prevalence and incidence in sub-Saharan Africa: A multi-level theoretical perspective. *American Journal of Community Psychology, 53*(1–2), 146–158. doi:10.1007/s10464-014-9628-4.

Wilson, J. (2009). Not so special after all? Daniels and the social determinants of health. *Journal of Medical Ethics, 35*, 3–6. doi:10.1136/jme.2008.024406.

World Bank. (2015a). *East Asia's changing urban landscape: Measuring a decade of spiritual growth.* Retrieved from http://www.worldbank.org/en/topic/urbandevelopment/publication/east-asias-changing-urban-landscape-measuring-a-decade-of-spatial-growth

World Bank. (2015b). *OVC Toolkit.* Retrieved from http://info.worldbank.org/etools/docs/library/162495/howknow/definitions.htm

World Health Organisation (WHO). (2003). *Social determinants of health. The solid facts. Second Edition.* Geneva: World Health Organization

World Health Organisation (WHO). (2006). *Constitution of the world health organization.* Basic Documents, Forty-fifth edition, Supplement, October 2006.

World Health Organisation (WHO). (2010a). *Tuberculosis fact sheet 104.* Retrieved from http://www.who.int/mediacentre/factsheets/fs104/en/print.html

World Health Organisation (WHO). (2010b). *Urban health equity assessment and response tool.* Retrieved from http://www.who.int/kobe_centre/measuring/urbanheart/en/

World Health Organisation (WHO). (2012). *Health behaviour in school- aged children (HBSC) study. International report from the 2009/2010 survey.* Retrieved from http://www.aim-digest.com/gateway/pages/S&P%20Alcohol%20and%20young%20People/Statistics/articles/HBSC.pdf

World Health Organisation (WHO). (2013). *HIV treatment guidelines.* Retrieved from http://www.who.int/hiv/pub/guidelines/arv2013/download/en/

World Health Organisation (WHO). (2014). *Consolidated guidelines on HIV prevention, diagnosis, treatment and care.* Retrieved from http://www.who.int/hiv/pub/guidelines/keypopulations/en/

World Health Organisation (WHO) & United Nations Human Settlements Programme (UN–Habitat). (2010). *Hidden cities unmasking and overcoming health inequities in urban settings.* Retrieved from http://www.who.int/kobe_centre/publications/hiddencities_media/who_un_habitat_hidden_cities_web.pdf?ua=1

Yankauer, A., Jr. (1950). The relationship of fetal and infant mortality to residential segregation: An inquiry into social epidemiology. *American Sociological Review, 15*(5), 644–648.

Zavaleta, D. (2007). *Missing dimensions of poverty data, the ability to go about without shame, a proposal for internationally comparable indicators of shame and humiliation* (OPHI Working Papers No. 3). Retrieved from http://www.ophi.org.uk/working-paper-number-03/

Ziraba, A. K., Madise, N., Mills, S., Kyobutungi, C., & Ezeh, A. (2009). Maternal mortality in the informal settlements of Nairobi city: What do we know? *Reproductive Health, 6*, 6. doi:10.1186/1742-4755-6-6.

Ziraba, A. K., Madise, N. J., Kimani, J. K., Oti, S., Mgomella, G., Matilu, M., & Ezeh, A. (2011a). Determinants for HIV testing and counselling in Nairobi urban informal settlements. *BioMed Centre, Public Health, 11*, 663.

Ziraba, A. K., Kyobutungi, C., & Zulu, E. M. (2011b). Fatal injuries in the slums of Nairobi and their risk factors: Results from a matched case–control study. *Journal of Urban Health, 88*(Suppl 2), 256–265. doi:10.1007/s11524-011-9580-7.

Zulu, E., Dodoo, F. N.-A., & Ezeh, A. C. (2002). Sexual risk-taking in the slums of Nairobi, Kenya, 1993–98. *Population Studies: A Journal of Demography, 56*(3), 311–323. doi:10.1080/00324720215933.

Zulu, E., Beguy, D., Ezeh, A. C., Bocquier, P., Madise, N. J., Cleland, J., & Falkingham, J. (2011). Overview of migration, poverty and health dynamics in Nairobi city's slum settlements. *Journal of Urban Health, 88*(2), 185–199. doi:10.1007/s11524-011-9595-0.

Chapter 3
HIV as an Urban Epidemic

Abstract HIV remains a major threat to life and livelihood and increasingly in urban contexts. This chapter presents the case of AIDS, globally, and the nature of vulnerability, risk and resilience against HIV in the urban spaces of Kenya and sub-Saharan Africa and describes the key populations most affected and infected by the virus.

Keywords HIV and AIDS • Ending AIDS • HIV global strategy • Key populations • Urban slums • Young people • Vulnerability • Risk • Resilience • Dignity and humiliation • Nairobi • Kenya

The Global AIDS Epidemic

The global HIV pandemic is in decline (UNAIDS 2014a). Since its inception, some 39 million people living with HIV have died (UNAIDS 2014a). From its peak in 2005, AIDS-related deaths have reduced by 35 per cent (UNAIDS 2014a). In 2013, worldwide, an estimated 1.5 million people died from AIDS-related causes compared to 2.4 million in 2005 (UNAIDS 2014a). New HIV infections have significantly fallen by around 38 per cent since 2001 (UNAIDS 2014d). An estimated 2.1 million people became newly infected with HIV in 2013, a reduction from 3.4 million in 2001 (UNAIDS 2014a). HIV infections among children in 2012 declined by 58 per cent since 2002 and 2013; 240,000 children became newly infected with HIV in 2013, a 40 per cent reduction since 2009 (UNAIDS 2014a).

By mid-2014, approximately 13.6 million people living with HIV had access to ART (UNAIDS 2014a). An estimated 38 per cent of all adults living with HIV were accessing treatment (UNAIDS 2014a). There is progress in providing antiretroviral

© The Author 2016

G. Jones, *HIV and Young People: Risk and Resilience in the Urban Slum*,
SpringerBriefs in Public Health, DOI 10.1007/978-3-319-26814-9_3

medicines to pregnant women living with HIV; in 2013, 67 per cent of pregnant women living with HIV in low- and middle-income countries were accessing ART, up from 47 per cent in 2010 (UNAIDS 2014a; UNICEF 2014). In sub-Saharan Africa, there was a decline between 2005 and 2013 in the number of reported AIDS-related deaths, falling by 39 per cent with new infections similarly reducing by 33 per cent for the same years (UNAIDS 2014a). Since 2009, there has been a 43 per cent decline in new HIV infections among children in the 21 priority countries of the Global Plan in Africa (UNAIDS 2014a).[1]

While noting the progress made, UNAIDS describes achievements as fragile (UNAIDS 2011). UNAIDS (2014a) estimates that of the 35 million people currently living with HIV, by the end of 2013, some 19 million did not know their HIV-positive status. In 2013, the global total of children under the age of 15 living with HIV was estimated at 3.2 million with only 24 per cent accessing ART (UNAIDS 2014a).

From the outset, sub-Sahara Africa has carried the heaviest AIDS burden. Up to 70 per cent of new HIV infections occurs in sub-Saharan Africa (UNAIDS 2014a). By the end of 2012, 71 per cent of the 35 million people living with HIV and 88 per cent of all children less than 15 years living with HIV were in sub-Saharan Africa (African Union 2013). More than 90 per cent of the global AIDS-related deaths among children under 15 years took place in sub-Saharan Africa (African Union 2013; UNAIDS 2013).

Currently there are an estimated 24.7 million people living with HIV in sub-Saharan Africa (UNAIDS 2014a). AIDS remains the leading cause of death throughout the last decade with 75 per cent of all AIDS-related deaths occurring in sub-Saharan Africa; in 2010, 1.8 million people died from AIDS-related illnesses (UNAIDS 2010b).

Three out of four people on ART live in sub-Saharan Africa (UNAIDS 2014a). For the subcontinent, while there are improvements in treatment coverage for people living with HIV, in 2013, 67 per cent of men and 57 per cent of women were not receiving ART in all countries of sub-Saharan Africa.

There is a strong gender dynamic to these statistics. In sub-Saharan Africa, women are disproportionately infected by HIV being twice more likely to acquire HIV via unprotected heterosexual sex than are men (UNAIDS 2014a). Of the almost 25 million people estimated to be living with HIV in sub-Saharan Africa, 58 per cent are women (UNAIDS 2014a). In sub-Saharan Africa, 25 per cent of all new infections are among adolescent girls and young women (UNAIDS 2014a). HIV is still a leading cause of death for women of reproductive age worldwide (UNAIDS 2014a).

---

[1] 'The Global Plan, 2012, is a multi-agency initiative established to work towards the elimination of new HIV infections among children by 2015 and keeping their mothers alive. The Global Plan prioritized 22 countries where 90 per cent of pregnant women living with HIV resided. Twenty-one of these countries are in sub Saharan Africa, of which Kenya is one' (UNAIDS 2014a).

There are marked differences within sub-Saharan Africa, with eastern and southern Africa claiming the heaviest toll for HIV and AIDS.[2] Combined, countries in this region account for an estimated 50 per cent of the global HIV burden (UNAIDS 2014e). However, progress in the region is noted with new HIV infections dropping by 32 per cent between 2005 and 2013 and over 8.1 million people from a total of 18.5 million living with HIV receiving treatment with the number of AIDS-related deaths for the same period falling by around 46 per cent (UNAIDS 2014e). Although there was significant scale up of services for mothers living with HIV through programmes targeting prevention of mother to child transmission (PMTCT) resulting in a reduction of 66 per cent of new infections among children, only 27 per cent of all children living with HIV were receiving ART (UNAIDS 2014e).

Of the more than 35 million people living with HIV, 4.2 million, or 15 per cent, reside in 30 cities in eastern and southern Africa (Van Renterghem et al. 2012). In sub-Saharan Africa, HIV prevalence is higher in urban areas than in rural settings; 30 of the 33 countries with the largest numbers of urban dwellers living with HIV are found in Nigeria, Zambia, Tanzania, Zimbabwe, Uganda and Kenya. Urban centres across eastern and southern Africa in particular are disproportionally affected by HIV (UNAIDS 2015). An association has been established between the degree of urbanisation and concentrations of HIV in all urban settings. This is predicted to intensify in the mid to long term (UNAIDS 2014c).

A Global Strategy to End AIDS

After three decades of HIV, a substantial body of knowledge has emerged on what needs to happen to end AIDS (UNAIDS 2011). The trajectory has been to move towards a people-centred and human rights-based approach that takes as its point of departure the multifaceted nature of discrimination, access and forms of vulnerability driving the disease (UNAIDS 2010a). In nearly all countries, national HIV strategic plans have been established and, especially in sub-Saharan Africa, managed by National AIDS Commissions,[3] which, for the better part, are comprehensive enough to guide concerted action to end AIDS.

---

[2] The countries of eastern and southern Africa are Angola, Botswana, Comoros, Eretria, Ethiopia, Kenya, Lesotho, Madagascar, Malawi, Mauritius, Mozambique, Namibia, Rwanda, Seychelles, South Africa, South Sudan, Swaziland, Tanzania, Uganda, Zimbabwe and Zambia (UNAIDS 2010b).

[3] The setting up of a National AIDS Commission and HIV strategic plan and tracking system is aligned to the 'Three Ones' principles applicable in all country-level HIV/AIDS response:

One agreed HIV/AIDS Action Framework that provides the basis for coordinating the work

of all partners; One National AIDS Coordinating Authority, with a broad based multi-sector mandate; and One agreed country-level Monitoring and Evaluation System (UNAIDS 2004).

In ending AIDS, the aspirational goal of UNAIDS is 'getting to zero'[4] (UNAIDS 2011). The objective is that the epidemic 'no longer represents a public health threat to any population or country…and that by 2030, the following targets have been reached: 90 per cent reduction in new infections; 90 per cent reduction in stigma and discrimination; 90 per cent reduction in AIDS related deaths' (UNAIDS 2014a, p.1)

To reach these targets, UNAIDS (2014b) highlights the primary importance of context and, in particular, location and population groups and advocates for an approach that essentially closes the gap between those who can access prevention and treatment and those who cannot. This approach realises that certain populations face a heightened vulnerability and are at increased risk of HIV infection, such as displaced HIV-positive young women and migrant groups. That is, to end AIDS, the gap between the most and least vulnerable to HIV infection needs to close (UNAIDS 2014b).

Key Populations at Higher Risk

An 'Investment Framework' was developed for ending AIDS. Based on existing evidence of what has been shown to work best in HIV prevention, treatment, care and support, it aims to facilitate a more focused and strategic use of scare resources (UNAIDS 2011). The Investment Framework cites a series of critical social and programmatic enablers essential to a prioritised AIDS response. As part of the goal of stopping new infections and keeping people alive, six programme activities are given in this framework, the first of which is a focus on key populations at higher risk, notably, sex workers and their clients, men who have sex with men and people who inject drugs (UNAIDS 2011). The list is not exhaustive as key populations differ according to context which, in turn, shapes the nature and scope of vulnerability to HIV infection. UNAIDS (2011) notes that the deeply embedded vulnerability of key populations disproportionately impacted by the epidemic has not changed in the face of urbanisation and the promise that it holds. However, the dynamic factors linked to this vulnerability and how they are subjectively defined and evaluated, certainly in the case of the urban slum, have not been comprehensively researched. Schwitters et al. (2015) argued that not all social groups equally benefit from the expansion of ART and other biomedical and behavioural interventions critical in slowing HIV transmission across sub-Saharan Africa. Populations at high risk of HIV infection, including men who have sex with men, sex workers and people who inject drugs, consistently face problems of access owing to structural factors, legal barriers, stigma and discrimination as well as remaining gaps in epidemiologic data on HIV prevalence and related behaviours. As such, much of these groups remain 'hidden populations' and continue to pose considerable challenges to research and population-based analysis.

---

[4] 'Zero new HIV infections; zero discrimination; and zero AIDS-related deaths' (UNAIDS 2011).

Urban-Based Sex Work

Drawing on global evidence, urban environments provide a greater range of opportunities for sexual mixing than other less concentrated settings (UNICEF 2012; 2013). In concentrated social environments, sexual mixing is facilitated by the Internet and mobile telephones, and particularly so for younger people. In urban settings, sexual connections are more likely to occur across social status and geographic location, including slum and non-slum areas. In the cash economy of the urban conurbation, disposable income more easily provides the option of paying for sex and liaisons for transactional sex[5] (UNICEF 2012; 2013).

Transactional relations based on the provision and payment for sex can include other forms of arrangements than payment of money, such as the provision of gifts (Maganja et al. 2007).

In sub-Saharan Africa, the evidence demonstrates that sex in exchange for material benefit occurs across a wide range of formal and informal relationships (Robinson and Yeh 2008). Opportunities for exchanging sex for money or other forms of trade are facilitated by population concentrations and the more liberal attitudes that characterise urban social life (Mberu 2012). Moore et al. (2007) state that within many high HIV prevalence countries, transactional sex reflects prevailing economic and social roles with men as providers of material benefits received by women. As MacPherson et al. (2012) demonstrated, given the power dynamics in relationships where women are less able to negotiate safer sex, there is always a greater chance of riskier sexual encounters. The context and motivation of engagement in different forms of transactional sex are critical in understanding risk and, in particular, perception of risk in these engagements. Based on a respondent-driven study of female sex workers in Nairobi, Musyoki et al. (2015) discovered that despite a high awareness of HIV among respondents, close to 60 per cent of all women remained unaware of their HIV-positive status, and almost half incorrectly believed they were HIV negative. Noting that HIV prevalence was 14 per cent among female sex workers between the ages of 18 and 24, this perception of invulnerability, borne partly out of age, increases the chances of transmitting HIV to both paying and non-paying partners and delays in accessing treatment and care interventions (Ministry of Public Health and Sanitation 2010).

Globally, sex workers have on average a 12 times higher ratio of HIV infection than for the adult population (UNAIDS 2014a). An underlying reason given is widespread violence and lack of redress involved in all forms of sex work (UNAIDS 2011). In a study of rape and client-initiated gender-based violence and associated risk among female sex workers in Kampala, Uganda, Schwitters et al. (2015) state that almost one-half of female sex workers reported having been raped at least once in their lifetime and 82 per cent had experienced client-initiated violence. In Kenya, the HIV prevalence rate for sex workers is estimated at 29.3 per cent (Ministry of Health et al. 2014). Drawing on information provided by two population-based HIV serologic surveys in Kenya in 2007 and 2008/2009, Musyoki et al. (2015) confirmed

---

[5] Transactional sex is discreet from formal sex work (MacPherson et al. 2012).

that the level of HIV infection among female sex workers is approximately three times that of women aged 15–49 years residing in Nairobi. Robinson and Yeh (2008) from a study in western Kenya showed that in all forms of sex work, providing higher costing risky sex helps cope with unanticipated shocks and stress factors that expose sex workers to a heightened risk of HIV infection. It is an instance of using a negative coping mechanism to answer an immediate threat that puts at risk long-term wellbeing. McKinnon et al. (2013) demonstrated that for Nairobi rates of prevalence were higher among male sex workers based on a survey of male sex workers in 'hot spots' across the city. Questions of vulnerability, humiliation and resilience among male sex workers are far less studied than that for female sex workers.

Available evidence suggests that urban-dwelling males are more likely to pay for sex than their rural counterparts (Pravin et al. 2014). Of the 23 countries with relevant survey data, slum-dwelling men in 15 countries demonstrated a higher propensity for purchasing sex than non-slum-dwelling men (Pravin et al. 2014). A case study in Tanzania shows that 9.5 per cent of slum-dwelling men paid for sex in the last year, compared with 3.6 per cent of non-slum-dwelling men (Pravin et al. 2014). The literature however is wanting in regard to the intra-urban dynamic of sex work. Moreover, the evidence is scant when it comes to women paying for sex, possibly revealing a gender bias in the research and a demonstration of assumptions relating to sexual behaviour in a patriarchal society (Pravin et al. 2014).

Musyoki et al. (2015) makes the point that studying young female sex workers perception towards risk and vulnerability poses many challenges stemming from the fact that behaviours associated with female sex workers are illegal and seen as immoral leading to significant degrees of stigmatisation; this is especially the case for probability-based surveys aimed at providing representative estimates of the biological and behavioural factors of female sex workers (Musyoki et al. 2015).

Men Who Have Sex With Men

Most marginalised groups, as illustrated by men who have sex with men (MSM), find protection in cities through the anonymity they afford (Human Science Research Council 2014). Spatial concentration also means that certain groups may find social and sexual networking easier. Social cohesion among all marginalised groups, especially MSM, varies remarkably and is majorly influenced by cultural attitudes towards and social acceptance of same-sex sexual behaviour, as well as the legal frameworks relevant to homosexuality (Human Science Research Council 2014). Living in an overwhelmingly hostile environment, MSM may seek safety in numbers with close proximity to likeminded people who provide invaluable social support (Human Science Research Council 2014).

Baral's data et al. (2012) indicates that MSM living in cities are more likely to acquire HIV than in other locations. Data from Nigeria shows that 25 per cent of MSM are living with HIV in Lagos, compared with 13.5 per cent of MSM nationally. In Kenya, although MSM are estimated to represent only 6 per cent of HIV infections in the largely rural Nyanza province, for example, they accounted for 16 per cent of new infections in Nairobi and more than 20 per cent in the urbanised coastal region (World Bank and UNAIDS 2009). Further study has given HIV-1 prevalence among MSM as very high in coastal areas of Kenya (Sanders et al. 2007).

Kennedy et al. (2013) studied MSM in urban centres in Swaziland and found that MSM face significant and multiple forms of stigma and discrimination related both to HIV status and sexual identity. Although violence was a common experience for MSM, given the criminalised nature of same-sex liaisons in the country, many MSM as a result of their sexuality did not bring reports of violence to the authorities (Kennedy et al. 2013). Stigma was reported as the predominant barrier to accessing health-care services for MSM living with HIV. Kennedy et al. (2013) reported that many MSM as a result of a stigmatised sexual identity (and disease) led to depression, self-stigma and shame. Poverty and lack of economic opportunities substantially shaped MSM risk-taking behaviours (Kennedy et al. 2013). In Swaziland, as elsewhere on the subcontinent and including Kenya, in principle, health services are available to all, yet there is a notable gap in HIV prevention services specifically tailored for MSM.

Injecting Drug Use

As Mathers et al. (2010) state, injection drug behaviours are long recognised as a key transmission route for HIV. Recent data shows an increase in injection drug use and associated HIV infections in sub-Saharan Africa (Mathers et al. 2010; Tun et al. 2015). From one study carried out in Nairobi, it was found that more than one-half of sexually active people who inject drugs (PWID) had non-injecting sex partners, a situation conducive for fuelling further the HIV epidemic in the general non-injecting population with PWID acting as a 'bridge population' (Gelmon et al. 2009). From a cross-sectional study carried out in Nairobi and supported by evidence elsewhere, it was shown that PWID face multiple accounts of stigma from the local community given the criminalised nature of their behaviour and being associated with multifarious criminal activity as many needed to engage in crime to support their addiction (DeBeck et al. 2007).

Urban centres routinely show a higher concentration of PWID (UNAIDS 2014c). A major reason for population concentration among PWID is that drugs of choice are more available in urban settings. A number of studies have found extremely high HIV prevalence among drug users in African cities (Brodish et al. 2011). Evidence drawn from Kenya and Tanzania indicated that injection drug use majorly contributed to the HIV epidemic in these and neighbouring countries (McCurdy et al. 2005).

Although there remains critical gaps in the evidence concerning injection drug use and associated HIV infections in Kenya, it is widely held that the use of injected heroin has gradually increased since the late 1990s notably with the availability of a higher and more concentrated form of heroin coming from Thailand.[6] As of late 2013, while the number of PWID was contested among researchers, the consensus

---

[6] 'Brown sugar', a lower grade of heroin, has been replaced by 'white crest' as did user habits shift from inhalation of the vapour from the former to the injecting of the latter (Beckerleg et al. 2006).

now puts the figure at between 6216 and 10,937 in Nairobi and 3718–8500 in the coastal area of Kenya (Kenya National AIDS & STI Control Programme (NASCOP) & Ministry of Health. (2013)). A recent study in Kenya estimated that HIV prevalence for PWID ranges between 20 and 50 per cent and that 80 per cent of PWID do not know their HIV status (Musyoki 2012). Most of these same PWID had reported low levels of education and were predominately men aged between 15 and 34 years (UNODC 2012). As Gouws et al. (2006) reported, compared with other key populations, PWID in Kenya remain a relatively small group, but note that HIV transmission through injection practices yield a far higher HIV incidence rate compared to transmission through heterosexual sex. Moreover, PWID have on average a two times higher probability of HIV transmission for each risky exposure compared to exposure from casual heterosexual sex (Gouws et al. 2006).

Kenya, HIV and the Urban Environment

Based on a combination of consistently high rates of morbidity and mortality, the HIV epidemic was considered a threat to Kenya's stability and future prosperity (British Broadcasting Company 1999); consequently, HIV was declared a national disaster. Although there have been substantial improvements in prevalence and incidence, HIV remains a major public health challenge.

Kenya is one of the six HIV 'high burden' countries in Africa (UNAIDS 2015). Out of a total population of 40 million, there are reckoned to be at least 1.6 million people currently living with HIV (NASCOP, NACC & UNAIDS 2014). Kenya has the second largest epidemic in eastern and southern Africa and the fourth largest globally (UNAIDS 2015). At the end of 2014, national HIV prevalence was estimated at 6 per cent and of all adults living with HIV, 58 per cent were women (NASCOP, NACC & UNAIDS 2014). Characterised by extreme heterogeneity, the epidemic in Kenya is considered 'mature' and generalised.[7] Nine counties in Kenya account for some 65 per cent of all new infections, which includes Nairobi County. Many of the highly burdened counties such as Nyanza in the west and Turkana in the north are classified as disaster prone and at times have been the scene for mass displacement and large-scale social upheaval resulting, very often, in rural to urban migration (NASCOP, NACC & UNAIDS 2014; United Nations Office for the Coordination of Humanitarian Affairs (OCHA) 2015).

In Kenya, as elsewhere in the region, the modes of transmission for HIV are diverse. The primary mode is sexual (NASCOP, NACC & UNAIDS 2014). HIV prevalence among key populations is estimated at 29.3 per cent for sex workers, 18.2 per cent for men who have sex with men and 18.3 per cent for injecting drug users (NASCOP, NACC & UNAIDS 2014). Declining from its peak in 2007, HIV prevalence has con-

---

[7] A concentrated HIV epidemic is when the rate of HIV is less than 1 per cent in the general population but more than 5 per cent in at least one high-risk subpopulation, such as MSM, IDUs, SW or their clients. A generalised HIV epidemic is when HIV prevalence rate exceeds 1 per cent in the general population (Denning 2014).

tinued to decline in Kenya with new infections stabilising at around 100,000 for the last decade (Carter 2014; Kimanga et al. 2014; NASCOP, NACC & UNAIDS 2014). In 2013, 21 per cent of new adult HIV infections occurred among young women aged 15–24 years. The rate of new infections per year exceeds the number of newly enrolled people on ART, put at 660,000 for both adults and children and frustrates attempts to control the national epidemic (NACC 2014). HIV-related deaths have reduced from 85,000 in 2006 to 58,000 in 2014 (NACC 2014). By the end of 2013, there were approximately 1.14 million orphans in Kenya as a result of AIDS-related deaths among parents and care givers, many of whom were born into or migrated to the urban slums (Ministry of Health, Kenya National AIDS Control Council (NACC) & National STI and AIDS Control Programme (NASCOP) (2014)). Nairobi City Council 2015).

The data shows considerable differences in HIV prevalence rates across location and socio-demographic groups. For example, Kimani-Murage et al. (2013) noted that according to the 2007 Kenya AIDS Indicator Survey, a higher proportion of people aged 15–64 years in urban areas (8.4 per cent) were infected with HIV, compared to those in rural areas (6.7 per cent). Women aged 15–49 years and urban residents are disproportionately burdened with HIV, compared to men and rural residents (Kenya National Bureau of Statistics and ICF Macro 2010; Ministry of Health, Kenya National AIDS Control Council (NACC) & National STI and AIDS Control Programme (NASCOP) (2014)). As APHRC report (2014), although the ratio has improved since 2000, women with no formal education continue to have the least knowledge of HIV and AIDS. Young slum-dwelling women, between the ages of 15 and 19, had the lowest proportion of testing for HIV, along with those in the category of never married (APHRC 2014).

Nairobi has a disproportionally high rate of HIV infection among slum-dwellers. Oti et al. (2013) argue that slum residents are more adversely affected by the HIV epidemic than non-slum residents since they generally exhibit worse health indicators than their non-slum-dwelling counterparts (Ross and Mirowsky 2001). From the time of the studies carried out by Lamba (1994) and UN-Habitat (2006b) on the impact of HIV in slum settlements in Kenya, there persist gaps in the information concerning the interplay of HIV vulnerability and risk in urban settings.

From the evidence of a 2008 seroprevalence study carried out in two slums in Nairobi based on a sample of 2000 adults aged 18 years and older, it showed a prevalence of 11.5 per cent, nearly double the national average and 1.5 times the prevalence for all of Nairobi city (Kenya National Bureau of Statistics and ICF Macro 2010; Oti et al. 2013). Similarly, from a comprehensive survey carried out in two Nairobi informal settlements by HIV prevalence , it was estimated at 12 per cent among slum-dwellers compared with 5 and 6 per cent among non-slum and rural residents, respectively (Madise et al. 2012). A similar trend was demonstrated by a 2005 household survey in Johannesburg, South Africa, which showed a far higher HIV prevalence in informal settlements, compared to formal urban settings (Vearey 2011).

The global picture concerning data from household surveys is obscure as to whether slum residence is associated with elevated HIV vulnerability; in many countries this is the case (UNAIDS 2014c). The reasons as to why the situation may be markedly different in cities of eastern and southern Africa remain unclear and to a degree a matter of conjecture. From the literature, in the case of Nairobi, the concentration of people living with HIV in slum communities is likely due to the depth of spiralling poverty and the presence of most vulnerable groups including migrant and marginalised populations. That is, the ever present magnitude of risk and lack of effective resilience act on each other and wholly diminish the range of options relating to health and healthy livelihoods. Whether this is owing fully or in part to the varying effect of humiliation felt by different population groups from varying cultural backgrounds is unknown.

Concerning knowledge of how to prevent HIV transmission, based on a cross-sectional slum survey, Mberu (2014) states, overall, slum-dwelling women demonstrate a higher knowledge compared not just to the rest of Nairobi but to Kenya as a whole. Furthermore, there is a notable increment in the knowledge among slum-dwelling inhabitants of HIV prevention strategies compared with the rest of Nairobi and Kenya (Mberu 2014). HIV testing in the slums in Nairobi demonstrated better indicators compared with other urban areas and the rest of Kenya (Mberu 2014). Given this added awareness, further research is required on the matter of perceiving resilience among slum-dwelling women given the consistently high rates of HIV incidence.

As Mberu says (2014), the correlation between adopting risk-reducing strategies and subjective perception of one's own risk is much discussed (Kohler et al. 2007; Smith 2003). Data from sub-Saharan Africa has shown a positive association between a correct assessment of risk regarding contracting an STI, including HIV, and deployment of protective behaviours, such as condom use (Mberu 2014). However, the question of self-evaluation of one's own risk and protective measures including behaviour change remains a highly contested subject and requires further investigation.

Treatment for HIV and AIDS

Following on from an announcement by the government of Kenya in 2006 that ART in all public hospitals and health centres is to be provided free of charge, national coverage increased significantly as part of the strategic plan to reach universal coverage Ministry of Health, Kenya National AIDS Control Council (NACC) & National STI and AIDS Control Programme (NASCOP) (2014). In 2010, WHO changed its treatment guidelines recommending an earlier start to ART, which had the effect of severely reducing the number of Kenyans receiving treatment (Kohler 2011; Ministry of Health, Kenya National AIDS Control Council (NACC) & National STI and AIDS Control Programme (NASCOP) (2014), Oti et al. 2013).[8]

Still, Oti et al. (2013) report strong improvement in HIV mortality as a result of 'going to scale' with ART provision in Kenya. HIV mortality decreased from 2.5

---

[8] According to the HIV treatment guidelines by the World Health Organization, ART is to be offered to all HIV-positive people at CD4 counts below 500 cells/mm, the previous WHO recommendation, set in 2010, was to offer treatment at a CD4 count of 350 or below (WHO 2013).

per 1000 persons at the outset of ART provision in 2003, when only 5 per cent of those needing ART were receiving it, to 1.7 per 1000 persons post-2006, when the risk of dying from HIV was 53 per cent less compared to the inception period (Oti et al. 2013). The decline in AIDS-related deaths occurred despite the still very high prevalence of HIV in slum settlements overall (Kyobutungi et al. 2008).

Women experienced a sharp decline in HIV mortality during this period, more than double the decline evidenced among men (Oti et al. 2013). Oti et al. (2013) add that the relatively wide-scale provision of free ART greatly assisted young people and women in particular. Since the advent of ART, there is evidence that HIV mortality has decreased significantly at the population level among Kenyan slum residents. However, in the slum areas studied, younger adults were more likely to be unemployed and hence less likely to afford treatment compared to older age groups. If the cost of medication was in reach, the associated costs, for example, transport and storage, may well prove prohibitive. The fact remains that even with noted treatment success, HIV remains a major cause of death among the urban poor as compared to other causes of mortality (Oti et al. 2013).

Perceived advantages of using ART may differ from one social group to another. Understanding the universe of the patient and subjective interpretation of associated benefits is critical to questions of vulnerability and resilience. One such assumption is that ART is taken simply to get well and can be understood in purely personal health terms, that is, the innate desire not to be ill. Drawing largely on anecdotal evidence from Nairobi, it is speculated that HIV prevention pills – post-exposure prophylaxis[9] – are used by sex workers in place of condoms so as to exact a higher payment from clients. However, in these cases, it is reported that the full course of PEP is rarely being followed and therefore allowing the possibility of drug resistance in the general public against antiretroviral medication (Gathura 2015). One conclusion to be drawn is the necessity for understanding the motivation for taking PEP and, possibly in the case of these sex workers, seeing it as a useful tool to combat disadvantage and discrimination, that is, a veritable means of resilience. Economic advantage in the short term leads to a greater chance of socioeconomic hardship in the long term. As discussed by Horstmann et al. (2010), a SMART programme takes account of all factors relevant to ART regimen adherence, which are invariably context driven. There is a difference in knowing what constitutes a SMART programme and seeing it realised by different social groups.

A body of evidence is emerging premised largely on qualitative research and now supported by quantitative data demonstrating that food insecurity is a major factor in poor ART adherence and particularly in resource-limited settings. Strategic information is still wanting, however, on the causal pathway between food insecurity and ART adherence, and further research is required which separates nutritional from household vulnerability. In a cross-sectional survey of people living with HIV on ART carried out in the city of Windhoek, Hong et al. (2014) state that four of the

---

[9] Post-exposure prophylaxis (PEP) is short-term antiretroviral treatment to reduce the likelihood of HIV infection after potential exposure either occupationally or through sexual intercourse (WHO 2013).

ten top reasons given for missing a medication dose were related to food insecurity and that severe household food insecurity was significantly associated with poor ART adherence (Hong et al. 2014). Without an adequate level of food and nutrition, the efficacy of ART is substantially reduced. Effective palliative care for HIV is based on nutritional needs being met, and as the evidences shows, all levels of malnutrition and wasting are linked to a poor response to antiretroviral treatment (Reynolds 2009). According to UN-Habitat (2011), the high cost of food for the urban poor can result in up to 70 per cent of household income being utilised to purchase food and not for other necessities such as schooling and health care.

In a study of selected Nairobi's slums, based on the Household Food Insecurity and Access Score, 65 per cent of households are now considered severely food insecure (Chaudhuri 2014). According to this Household Hunger Scale, 12 per cent of households are severely hungry and 37 per cent experience moderate hunger, and nutrition data reveal that 7500 children suffer from severe and acute malnutrition (Chaudhuri 2014). The evidence points to a deteriorating situation in Nairobi's slums in regard to higher rates of food insecurity and decline in dietary diversity (Chaudhuri 2014).

References

African Population and Health Research Center. (2014). *Population and health dynamics in Nairobi's informal settlements. Report of the Nairobi Cross-sectional Slums Survey (NCSS) 2012*. Nairobi: African Population and Health Research Center.

African Union. (2013, December 30). *Second desk review/popular version: Women and girls, HIV/ AIDS and conflicts: Situation analysis of 11 selected conflict and post- conflict countries in Africa*. Retrieved from http://www.aidswatchafrica.org/sites/default/files/publication-documents/2nd%20Desk%20Review%20Popular%20Report%20final%20copy.pdf

Beckerleg, S., Telfer, M., & Sadiq, A. (2006). A rapid assessment of heroin use in Mombasa, Kenya. *Substance Use and Misuse, 41*(6–7), 1029–1044.

British Broadcasting Company. (1999, November 26). AIDS declared a national emergency. *BBC News*. Retrieved from http://news.bbc.co.uk/2/hi/africa/538071.stm

Brodish, P., Singh, K., Rinyuri, A., Njeru, C., Kingola, C., Mureithi, P., Sambisa, W., & Weir, S. (2011). Evidence of high-risk sexual behaviors among injection drug users in the Kenya PLACE study. *Drug and Alcohol Dependence, 119*(1–2), 138–141. doi:10.1016/j.drugalcdep.2011.05.030.

Carter, M. (2014, February 17). HIV prevalence and incidence fall in Kenya. *Nam-AIDSMap*. Retrieved from http://www.aidsmap.com/HIV-prevalence-and-incidence-fall-in-Kenya/page/2827600/

Chaudhuri, J. (2014). *Indicator development for the surveillance of urban emergencies (IDSUE)* (Year 3 Research Report, August 2012 – December 2013). Nairobi: USAID.

DeBeck, K., Shannon, K., Wood, E., Li, K., Montaner, J., & Kerr, T. (2007). Income generating activities of people who inject drugs. *Drug and Alcohol Dependence, 91*(1), 50–56. doi:10.1016/j.drugalcdep.2007.05.003.

Denning, P. D. (2014). *Communities in crisis: Is there a generalized HIV epidemic in impoverished urban areas of the United States?* Retrieved from: http://www.cdc.gov/hiv/risk/other/poverty.html

Gathura, G. (2015, February 5). Sex workers using ARVs to charge clients more. *The Standard Digital News*. Retrieved from http://www.standardmedia.co.ke/health/article/2000150544/sex-workers-using-arvs-to-charge-clients-more

Gelmon, L., Kenya, P., Oguya, F., Cheluget, B., & Hailee, G. (2009). *Investing in children and youth: A World Bank strategy to fight poverty, reduce inequality and promote human development*. Washington, DC: World Bank.

Gouws, E., White, P. J., Stover, J., & Brown, T. (2006). Short term estimates of adult HIV incidence by modes of transmission: Kenya and Thailand as examples. *Journal of Sexually Transmitted Infections, 82*(3), 51–55. doi:10.1136/sti.2006.020164.

Hong, S. Y., Fanelli, T. J., Jonas, A., Gweshe, J., Tjituka, F., Sheehan, H. M., Wanke, C., Terrin, N., Jordan, M. R., & Tang, A. M. (2014). Household food security associated with antiretroviral therapy adherence among HIV-infected patients in Windhoek, Namibia. *Journal of Acquire Immune Deficiency Syndrome, 67*(4), 115–122. doi:10.1097/QAI.0000000000000308.

Horstmann, E., Brown, J., Islam, F., Buck, J., & Agins, B. D. (2010). Retaining HIV- infected patients in care: Where are we? Where do we go from here? *Oxford Journal of Medicine & Health, Clinical Infectious Disease, 50*(5), 752–761. doi:10.1086/649933.

Human Science Research Council. (2014). *Three cities study: High levels of HIV infection found among men who have sex with men (HIV/AIDS, STI and TB)*. Retrieved from http://www.hsrc.ac.za/en/research-outputs/view/7137.

Joint United Nations Programme on HIV/AIDS (UNAIDS). (2004, November 23). *Women and AIDS: A growing challenge* (Fact Sheet), Retrieved from http://data.unaids.org/Publications/Fact-Sheets04/fs_women_en.pdf

Joint United Nations Programme on HIV/AIDS (UNAIDS). (2010a). *UNAIDS 2011–2015 strategy getting to zero*. Geneva: UNAIDS.

Joint United Nations Programme on HIV/AIDS (UNAIDS). (2010b). *Global report: UNAIDS report on the global AIDS epidemic*. Geneva: UNAIDS.

Joint United Nations Programme on HIV/AIDS (UNAIDS). (2011). *A new investment framework for the global HIV response* (UNAIDS Issues Brief). Geneva: UNAIDS.

Joint United Nations Programme on HIV/AIDS (UNAIDS). (2013). *Global epidemic*. Geneva: UNAIDS.

Joint United Nations Programme on HIV/AIDS (UNAIDS). (2014a). *UNAIDS briefing book July 2014*. Geneva: UNAIDS.

Joint United Nations Programme on HIV/AIDS (UNAIDS). (2014b). *The gap report*. Geneva: UNAIDS.

Joint United Nations Programme on HIV/AIDS (UNAIDS). (2014c). *The cities report*. Retrieved from http://issuu.com/pm.dstaids.sp/docs/jc2687_thecitiesreport_en

Joint United Nations Programme on HIV/AIDS (UNAIDS). (2014d). *World AIDS day 2014, Fact sheet*. Retrieved from http://www.unaids.org/en/resources/campaigns/world-AIDS-Day-Report-2014/factsheet

Joint United Nations Programme on HIV/AIDS (UNAIDS). (2014e). *Eastern and Southern Africa HIV epidemic profile*. Retrieved from http://www.unaidsrstesa.org/wp-content/uploads/2015/06/unaids_profile_Regional.pdf

Joint United Nations Programme on HIV/AIDS (UNAIDS). (2015). UNAIDS regional support team for Eastern and Southern Africa. Retrieved from http://www.unaidsrsstesa.org/region/region-profile

Kennedy, C. E., Baral, S. D., Fielding-Miller, R., Adams, D., Dludlu, P., Sithole, B., Fonner, V. A., Mnisi, Z., & Kerrigan, D. (2013). "They are human beings, they are Swazi": Intersecting stigmas and the positive health, dignity and prevention needs of HIV-positive men who have sex with men in Swaziland. *Journal of International AIDS Society, 16*(4 Suppl 3), 18749. doi:10.7448/IAS.16.4.18749.

Kenya National AIDS Control Council (NACC). (2014). *Kenya AIDS response progress report 2014, progress towards zero*. Retrieved from http://www.unaids.org/sites/default/files/en/dataanalysis/knowyourresponse/countryprogressreports/2014ountries/KEN_narrative_report_2014.pdf

Kenya National AIDS & STI Control Programme (NASCOP) & Ministry of Health. (2013). *Kenya most at risk population size estimate consensus report*. Retrieved from

Kenya National Bureau of Statistics (KNBS) and ICF Macro. (2010). *Kenya demographic and health survey 2008–09*. Calverton: KNBS and ICF Macro.

Kenya National AIDS & STI control Programme (NASCOP), & Kenya National AIDS Control Council (NACC) & Joint United Nations Programme on HIV/AIDS (UNAIDS). (2014). *HIV/ AIDS in Kenya 2014 fact sheet.*

Kimanga, D. O., Ogola, S., Umuro, M., Ng'ang'a, A., Kimondo, L., Murithi, P., Muttunga, J., Waruiru, W., Mohammed, I., Sharrif, S., De Cock, K. M., Kim, A. A., & KAIS Study Group. (2014). Prevalence and incidence of HIV infection, trends, and risk factors among persons aged 15–64 years in Kenya: Results from a nationally representative study. *Journal of Acquired Immune Deficiency Syndrome, 1*(66 Suppl 1), 13–26. doi:10.1097/QAI.0000000000000124.

Kimani-Murage, E. W., Kyobutungi, C., Ezeh, A. C., Wekesah, F., Wanjohi, M., Muriuki, P., Musoke, R. N., Norris, S. A., Griffiths, P., & Madise, N. J. (2013). Effectiveness of person-alised, home-based nutritional counselling on infant feeding practices, morbidity and nutritional outcomes among infants in Nairobi slums: Study protocol for a cluster randomised controlled trial. *Trials, 14,* 445. doi:10.1186/1745-6215-14-445.

Kohler, P. K. (2011). Implementation of free cotrimoxazole prophylaxis improves clinic retention among ART-ineligible clients in Kenya. *AIDS, 25*(13), 1657–1661. doi:10.1097/ QAD.0b013e32834957fd.

Kohler, H. P., Behrman, J. R., & Watkins, S. C. (2007). Social networks and HIV/AIDS risk perceptions. *Demography, 44*(1), 1–33. doi:10.1353/dem.2007.0006.

Kyobutungi, C., Ziraba, A. K., Ezeh, A., & Yé, Y. (2008). *The burden of disease profile of residents of Nairobi's slums: Results from a demographic surveillance.* doi:10.1186/1478-7954-6-1.

Lamba, D. (1994). The forgotten half; environmental health in Nairobi's poverty areas. *Environment and Urbanization, 6,* 164–168.

MacPherson, E. E., Sadalaki, J., Njoloma, M., Nyongopa, V., Nkhwazi L., Mwapasa V., Lalloo, D. G., Desmond, N., Seeley, J., & Theobald, S. (2012). Understanding the gendered structural drivers of HIV in fishing communities in Southern Malawi. *Journal of the International AIDS Society, 15*(1), 1–9. doi:http://dx.doi.org/10.7448/IAS.15.3.17364.

Madise, N. J., Ziraba, A. K., Inungu, J., Khamadi, S. A., Ezeh, A., Zulu, E. M., Kebaso, J., Okoth, V., & Mwau, M. (2012). Are slum dwellers at heightened risk of HIV infection than other urban residents? Evidence from population-based HIV prevalence surveys in Kenya. *Health & Place, 18*(5), 1144–1152. doi:10.1016/j.healthplace.2012.04.003.

Maganja, R. K., Maman, S., Groves, A., & Mbwambo, J. K. (2007). Skinning the goat and pulling the load: Transactional sex among youth in Dar es Salaam, Tanzania. *AIDS Care: Psychological and Socio-medical Aspects of AIDS/HIV, 19*(8), 974–981. doi:10.1080/ 09540120701294286.

Mathers, B. M., Degenhardt, L., Ali, H., Wiessing, L., Hickman, M., Mattick, R. P., Myers, B., Ambekar, A., & Strathdee, S. A. (2010). *HIV prevention, treatment and care services for people who inject drugs: A systematic review of global, regional, and national coverage, 2009* (Reference Group to the United Nations on HIV and injecting drug use). *The Lancet, 375*(9719), 1014–1028. doi:http://dx.doi.org/10.1016/S0140-6736(10)60232-2.

Mberu, B. U. (2012, November 11). *Adolescent sexual and reproductive health and rights: Research evidence from sub-Saharan Africa.* PPD conference "Evidence for action: South-south collaboration for ICPD beyond 2014," Ruposhi Bangla Hotel, Dhaka. Abstract retrieved from http://r4d.dfid.gov.uk/PDF/Outputs/StepUp/2012_PPDMberu.pdf

Mberu, B. U. (2014). HIV/AIDS and other sexually transmitted infections. (Chapter 9). In African Population and Health Research Center (Ed.), *Population and health dynamics in Nairobi's informal settlements. Report of the Nairobi Cross-sectional Slums Survey (NCSS) 2012.* Nairobi: African Population and Health Research Center.

McCurdy, S. A., Williams, M. L., Ross, M. W., & Kilonzo, G. P. (2005). New injecting practice increases HIV risk among drug users in Tanzania. *British Medical Journal, 331*(7519), 778. doi:10.1136/bmj.331.7519.778-a.

McKinnon, L. R., Gakii, G., Juno, J. A., Izulla, P., Munyao, J., Ireri, N., Kariuki, C. W., Shaw, S. Y., Nagelkerke, N. J. D., Gelmon, L., Musyoki, H., Muraguri, N., Kaul, R., Lorway, R., & Kimani, J. (2013). High HIV risk in a cohort of male sex workers from Nairobi, Kenya. *Sexually Transmitted Infestations.* doi:10.1136/sextrans-2013-051310.

Ministry of Health, Kenya National AIDS Control Council (NACC) & National STI and AIDS Control Programme (NASCOP). (2014). *Kenya HIV prevention revolution road map: Count down to 2030*. Nairobi: National AIDS Control Council.

Ministry of Public Health and Sanitation. (2010). *National guidelines for HIV/STI programs for sex workers*. Retrieved from www.nascop.or.ke

Moore, A. M., Biddlecom, A. E., & Zulu, E. M. (2007). Prevalence and meanings of exchange of money or gifts for sex in unmarried adolescent sexual relationships in sub Saharan Africa. *African Reproductive Health, 11*, 44–61. Retrieved from http://www.ncbi.nlm.nih.gov/pubmed/18458736

Musyoki, H. (2012). *MARPS and vulnerable groups program*. Nairobi: National AIDS/STI Control Programme.

Musyoki, H., Kellogg, T. A., Geibel, S., Muraguri, N., Okal, J., Tun, W., Fisher Raymond, H., Dadabhai, S., Sheehy, M., & Kim, A. A. (2015). Prevalence of HIV, sexually transmitted infections, and risk behaviours among female sex workers in Nairobi, Kenya. *AIDS Behaviour, 19*(1), 46–58. doi:10.1007/s10461-014-0919-4.

Nairobi City Council/County Helath Services (2015). Nairobi City County Response to the HIV Epidemic. Unpublished raw data.

Oti, S. O., Mutua, M., Mgomella, G. S., Egondi, T., Ezeh, E., & Kyobutungi, C. (2013). HIV mortality in urban slums of Nairobi, Kenya 2003–2010: A period effect analysis. *BMC Public Health, 13*, 588. doi:10.1186/1471-2458-13-588.

Pravin, K. J., Sahu D. K., Reddy, S., Narayan, P., & Pandey, A. (2014). Multiple sexual partners and vulnerability to HIV: A study of patterns of sexual behaviour in the slum population of India. *World Journal of AIDS*. doi:http://dx.doi.org/10.4236/wja.2014.44044.

Reynolds, L. (2009). *Nutrition in ART programmes*. Retrieved from AIDSMap website: http://www.aidsmap.com/Nutrition-in-ART-programmes/page/1325010/

Robinson, J., & Yeh, E. (2008). *Transactional sex as a response to risk in western Kenya* (MPRA_paper_7405). Retrieved from http://mpra.ub.uni-muenchen.de/7405/

Ross, C. E., & Mirowsky, J. (2001). Neighborhood Disadvantage, Disorder and Health.*Journal of Health and Social Behavior, 42*(3),258–276. Retrieved from http://www.jstor.org/stable/3090214.

Sanders, E. J., McGraham, S., Okuku, H. S., van der Elst, E. M., Muhaari, A., Davies, A., Peshu, N., Price, M., McClelland, R. S., & Smith, A. D. (2007). HIV-1 infection in high risk men who have sex with men in Mombasa, Kenya. *AIDS, 21*(18), 2513–2520. doi:10.1097/QAD.0b013e3282f70a.

Schwitters, A., Lederer, P., Zilversmit, L., Gudoc, P. S., Ramiroe, I., Cumba, L., Mahagaja, E., & Jobarteh, K. (2015). Barriers to health care in rural Mozambique: A rapid ethnographic assessment of planned mobile health clinics for ART. *Global Health: Science and Practice, 3*(1), 109–116. doi:10.9745/GHSP-D-14-00145.

Smith, D. J. (2003). Imagining HIV/AIDS: Morality and perceptions of personal risk in Nigeria. *Journal of Medical Anthropology, 22*(4), 343–372. doi:10.1177/004208168702300206.

Tun, W., Sheehy, M., Broz, D., Okal, J., Muraguri, N., Raymond, H. F., Musyoki, H., Andrea, A. K., Muthui, M., & Geibel, S. (2015). HIV/STI prevalence and injection behaviors among people who inject drugs in Nairobi: Results from a 2011 bio-behavioral study using respondent-driven sampling. *AIDS and Behaviour, 19*(1 Suppl), 24–35. doi:10.1007/s10461-014-0936-3.

United Nations Office on Drugs and Crime (UNODC). (2012). *World Drug Report 2012*. Retrieved from http://www.unodc.org/unodc/en/data-and-analysis/WDR-2012.html.

United Nations Children's Fund (UNICEF). (2012). *State of the world's children. Children in an urban world*. Retrieved from http://www.unicef.org/sowc2012/

United Nations Children's Fund (UNICEF). (2013). *Towards an AIDS-free generation. Sixth stock-taking report*. Retrieved from http://www.unicef.org/publications/index_70986.html

United Nations Children's Fund (UNICEF). (2014). *Wide political support for eliminating 90 % of new HIV infections in children is yielding impressive results*. Retrieved from http://www.unicef.org/publications/index_51775.html

United Nations Human Settlements Programme (UN–Habitat). (2006a). *Nairobi: Urban sector profile.* Retrieved from http://unhabitat.org/

United Nations Human Settlements Programme (UN–Habitat). (2006b). *State of the world's cities 2006/7. Human settlements programme: The millenium development goals and urban sustainability-30 years of shaping the Habitat agenda.* Retrieved from http://www.amazon.com/State-Worlds-Cities-2006-Sustainability/dp/1844073785

United Nations Human Settlements Programme (UN–Habitat). (2011). *23rd Governing Council of UN-Habitat.* Retrieved from http://unhabitat.org/

United Nations Office for the Coordination of Humanitarian Affairs (UN/OCHA). (2015). *Kenya Humanitarian Overview.* Retrieved from https://fts.unocha.org/pageloader.aspx?page=emerg-emergencyCountryDetails&cc=ken

Van Renterghem, H., Colvin, M., de Beer, I., Gunthorp, J., Odii, M., Thomas, L., Jackson, H., & Getahun, M. (2012). *The urban HIV epidemic in Eastern and Southern Africa: Need for better KYE/KYR to inform adequate city responses.* Paper presented at the XIX international AIDS conference, Washington DC Conference, 2010, July 22–27. Abstract retrieved from http://pag.aids2012.org/EPosterHandler.axd?aid=16308UNDP

Vearey, J. (2011). Challenging urban health: Towards an improved local government response to migration, informal settlements, and HIV in Johannesburg, South Africa. *Global Health Action, 4.* doi:10.3402/gha.v4i0.5898.

World Bank & Joint United Nations Programme on HIV/AIDS (UNAIDS) Kenya. (2009). *HIV prevention response and modes of transmission analysis.* Retrieved from http://www.unaidsrstesa.org/sites/default/files/modesoftransmission/kenya_Mot_country_synthesis_report_22Mar09.pdf

World Health Organisation (WHO). (2013). *HIV treatment guidelines.* Retrieved from http://www.who.int/hiv/pub/guidelines/arv2013/download/en/

Chapter 4
Young People: Vulnerability, Risk and HIV in the Urban Slum

Abstract This chapter reviews the major literature on youth vulnerability to HIV in the urban slum and explores the key dynamic of gender and gender relations.

Keywords HIV • Urban slum settlements • Adolescents • Self-perception and risky behaviour • Poverty • Gender • Vulnerability • Resilience • Dignity and humiliation • Kenya

Adolescence and Risk

Nearly half of the global population is under the age of 25, the largest generation of children and youth in history, and close to 90 per cent of all young people live in the developing world (Canadian International Development Agency 2014). As Resnick and Casale (2014) point out, in sub-Saharan Africa, the 'youth bulge' refers to the fact that 60 per cent of the population are under the age of 25. According to UNICEF (2012), more than one billion children live in urban areas, and on average, young people account for 60 per cent of all people living in urban areas in low- and middle-income countries. By 2030, it is projected that up to 60 per cent of all urban dwellers will be under the age of 18 (UNICEF 2012). From demographic records (UN-Habitat 2014b), the data demonstrates that the population of sub-Saharan Africa is youthful with an increasing number born into or migrating to urban slums. Emina et al. (2011) have shown (and corroborated by Kabiru et al. 2013) that in many of the slums of Nairobi, over 30 per cent of the population is under the age of 15, with a further 22 per cent aged 15–24 years. As Cotton points out (2013), unlike other epochs in history, urbanisation in sub-Saharan Africa during the twentieth century did not bring with it far reaching economic and social improvements.

© The Author 2016

G. Jones, *HIV and Young People: Risk and Resilience in the Urban Slum*,
SpringerBriefs in Public Health, DOI 10.1007/978-3-319-26814-9_4

Young people growing up in urban slums can be extremely vulnerable (Kabiru et al. 2013). It is widely argued that this vulnerability is rooted in deprivation, poverty and powerlessness on their part or that of the primary caregivers to affect their situations (United Nations Children's Fund UNICEF 2012). Much of the literature points to growing up in ramshackle dwellings and overcrowded settlements with the constant fear of eviction and likely homelessness. In a UN-Habitat report (2013a), lack of suitable shelter and sanitation is the most pressing needs facing children in urban slums given that overcrowded conditions, lack of ventilation and inadequate natural light lead to a range of chronic ailments. Significant disparities in nutritional status have been noted for children living in 'rich' and 'poor' urban centres (UNICEF 2012). Children living in informal urban settlements are particularly vulnerable to child mortality before the age of 5; an indicator that is closely tied to extreme poverty and inadequate services (UNICEF 2012). Based mostly on research carried out in Asian cities, children and especially orphans and street children[1] are also particularly at risk of facing violence and abuse in urban slums (UNICEF 2012). Based on data taken from 80 less developed countries between 1990 and 2005 on under-5 mortality, Jorgensen and Rice (2012) argue that a consequence of the contextual and dynamic in urban slums is the social reproduction of child mortality.

The World Bank (2015a, b) has pointed to the fact that while all children are vulnerable, some are far more vulnerable than others. Under the age of majority (18), a most vulnerable child is at high risk of lacking adequate care and protection. With each new shock experienced directly and/or to the primary caregiver, a new level of vulnerability and risk emerges, and child vulnerability becomes a downward spiral (World Bank 2015b). Few studies, however, have looked at the lifetime effects that the slum has on children's psychological development, notably, the means of protection and security critical for social and cognitive development during early life. Research on vulnerable children in the slums of sub-Saharan Africa has been skewed, and as a result, more needs to be known about the specific detail of vulnerability and subjective perception at any one time. When data on the situation of children living in urban poverty is disaggregated, it reveals that this population group is largely absent from 'action research' and notably so in sub-Saharan Africa, with the result that the web of vulnerabilities faced by children and young people are inadequately captured and fail to inform policy and appropriate service delivery.

Young people are especially infected and affected by HIV (UNAIDS 2014). Young women have a heightened chance of experiencing gender-based violence than older women, and the link between all forms of sexual violence and HIV has

---

[1] '"Street children" is a term often used to describe both *market children* (who work in the streets and markets of cities selling or begging, and live with their families) and homeless street children (who work, live and sleep in the streets, often lacking any contact with their families). At highest risk is the latter group. Murder, consistent abuse and inhumane treatment are the "norm" for these children, whose ages range from 6 to 18. They often resort to petty theft and prostitution for survival. They are extremely vulnerable to sexually transmitted diseases including HIV/AIDS…' (Mexico Child Link 2003).

been documented (Anderson et al. 2008; UNAIDS 2014). The basis for young people's vulnerability to HIV is premised on the structural, social and behavioural dynamics which include lack of youth employment opportunities linked to conditions of enduring poverty and a sense of hopelessness linked to substance abuse (Anderson et al. 2008). Of the studies that look directly at HIV vulnerability among youth in slum settings, it was largely found that young people experienced increased vulnerability in the urban slum due to high-risk sexual behaviour, which has to be considered in the context of culture, gender, mobility, migration and displacement (Kabiru et al. 2013; Muindi et al. 2014). Data has shown that young people, more than any other age group, engage in behaviours that place them at greater risk of HIV. The 15–24 age group accounts for 39 per cent of all new HIV infections, and half of all HIV infections occur before the age of 25 (UNAIDS 2014). According to UNAIDS (2014), there are currently an estimated 2.1 million adolescents living with HIV; in sub-Saharan Africa, 60 per cent of all adolescents living with HIV are girls. Many of these adolescents are urban, do not know their HIV status and, in the absence of ART, are extremely vulnerable to poor health and face the constant risk of being ostracised from significant others including peers.

High-Risk Sexual Behaviour

The literature agrees that a key measure of vulnerability to HIV infection is age of sexual debut, which reflects local cultural practices and attitudes towards sexual relations, especially concerning young people. Research carried out in South Africa has broadly found that young people aged 12–24 in informal urban settlements have the highest rates of sexual experience nationwide and that for men it is influenced by status seeking and construction of identity in that environment (Gibbs et al. 2014). Hapern and Haydon (2012), however, estimate that although, globally, sexual activity begins for a quarter of all adolescents below the age of 15, sexual debut occurs later among urban dwellers than their rural counterparts and suggests that a major reason is a move away from early marriage in urban contexts – aggregating both slum and non-slum areas. In their study of male adolescents in Brazil's 'favelas', Juarez and Martin (2006) found that early sexual initiation was a discernible pattern, with nearly two-thirds of adolescents reporting first sex before age 15 and 17 per cent before age 13. Looking at unintended pregnancies among adolescents in Nairobi's slums, Mumah et al. (2014) found that slum-based adolescents were more likely to report earlier sexual activity earlier and sex work, unprotected sex and multiple sexual partnerships, compared with adolescents in non-slum areas. By age 16, 40 per cent of adolescent young women in Kenya's slums are sexually experienced, compared with 20 per cent of the general population (Mumah et al. 2014). According to Mberu (2008), the dual and interrelated indicator relevant in understanding sexual behaviour and reproductive health is the age of first sexual encounter and whether a condom was used. In short, if a condom was used for the first sexual episode, then further use is likely (Abma and Mcgill 2007; Shafil et al. 2004).

Research into adolescent sexual behaviour in slum settings reveals that condom use is low, in keeping with the broader trend of low condom use among adolescents in general. Although there is an urban advantage with respect to condom use, regular use of condoms among adolescents is generally found to be low in all settings. UNICEF (2010) reports that among adolescents, condom use among young women is consistently lower than among boys of the same age. The low level of condom use at premarital sexual initiation in Nigeria (15.8 per cent) is comparable to low prevalence among youths in most countries of sub-Saharan Africa, for example, 15 per cent in Tanzania, Malawi and Ethiopia (William and Alexander 1999) and 15.2 per cent in Angola (Ndola et al. 2005). However, these rates are lower compared to Lesotho (34 per cent for men and 59 per cent for women), Uganda (43 per cent for men) and Ghana (18 per cent for men and 27 per cent for women) (Tumwesigye et al. 2005).

In a study on sexual and reproductive health of adolescents in urban slums in Kenya, Beguy et al. (2013) found that condom use was overwhelmingly low among adolescents for their first sexual encounter due primarily to lack of knowledge. Among sexually experienced 12–14 year olds, none of the males and only 15 per cent of females reported using a condom at their first encounter. Condom use at last intercourse was nearly twice as high among males (46 per cent) compared with their female counterparts (24 per cent). Mumah et al. (2014) also found low rates of condom use for young men and young women – 29 and 26 per cent, respectively – between the ages of 12 and 22 in Nairobi slums for first sexual encounters. In that study, reasons given for risky sexual behaviour include poor parent-child communication on safe sex, lack of parental presence and weak family ties. In their study of condom use among adolescent males in Brazil's favelas, Juarez and Martin (2006) report that key barriers to condom use include clinic opening hours – clinics are generally closed at night and on weekends – and lack of planning ahead among adolescents so that they are not able to obtain a condom when needed.

Juarez and Martin (2006) also explored the sexual lives of adolescent boys in relation to condom use. The early period of sexual learning and experimentation during adolescence is often characterised by short-term relationships and relatively frequent partner change – in other words, rapid serial monogamy. Although the dominant pattern is of serial monogamy, 36 per cent of adolescent boys reported having ever had multiple partners at the same time, and 53 per cent of participants reported that their last sexual encounter took place within the context of casual relationships. Condoms are often associated with casual sex, promiscuity, infidelity and disease. In the context of a romantic relationship, proposing condom use may be interpreted as an admission or accusation of sexual infidelity (Gavin 2000). The conclusion reached based on the empirical evidence is that condom use as a habitual component of adolescent sexual activity is highly inconsistent and 'unprotected' sex still common.

In their study of female adolescents in Nairobi's slums, Mumah et al. (2014) found that peer pressure exposed adolescents to early sexual initiation and encouraged them to stay sexually active and to be seen to be doing so by their peers. Particularly for young women, the need to conform and stand out among peers had a strong bearing on choices related to sexual activity (Norr et al. 2004). For boys, sexual activity was seen as the core of their masculinity. Conversely, boys without a sexual partner experienced disrespect and risked alienation among peers (Mumah et al. 2014). In the Mumah et al. (2014) study, findings showed that for both boys and young women, there was the threat of being stigmatised if a desire to use a contraceptive was expressed. In a separate study, familial influence was also seen as impacting age of sexual debut among young women in Nairobi's slums, with adolescent young women 42 per cent less likely to have ever had sex when the father is present in the household (Ngom et al. 2003). The conclusion drawn is that in the slums of Nairobi, father's presence, unlike that of the mother, is associated with a stronger sense of resilience during adolescence (Ngom et al. 2003).

Poverty and Material Deprivation

Mumah et al. (2014) tied high-risk sexual behaviour and adverse sexual and reproductive health outcomes to, in part, the numerous socioeconomic and health challenges that adolescents face in their communities. These include insecurity from high levels of crime and violence and overwhelming impoverishment. In their study of sexual and reproductive health of adolescents in urban slums in Kenya, Beguy et al. (2013) corroborate the findings that adolescents constitute approximately 30 per cent of the total slum population and are at special risk of extreme poverty and associated factors of early marriage, illiteracy, sexual abuse and lack of access to essential services. Impacted by these factors, young people face a greater chance of HIV infection and early childbearing.

Similarly, Kamndaya et al. (2014) followed up on Greif (2012) by looking at the relationship between material deprivation and sexual risk behaviours among adolescents in urban slums in South Africa. They found that material deprivation – unmet needs of housing, food and health care – was significantly associated with increased odds of high sexual risk-taking for young men and young women in the urban slum. Financial difficulty was the major motivation for sexual risk-taking of young women, in particular. In South Africa's urban slums, a large proportion of slum residents live without access to basic services, and both HIV prevalence and incidence are much higher in these settings. One in five residents is estimated to be living with HIV, and just under a third of new infections occur in slum areas every year (Kamndaya et al. 2014). The results support the idea that environment has not been adequately taken into account in understanding and responding to HIV risk factors in slum settings and that findings need further analysis regarding different population groups, including long-term residents and recent arrivals into the slum.

Mugisha et al. (2003) looked at alcohol, substance and drug use among urban slum adolescents in Nairobi and noted the connection between these risky behaviours and economic deprivation. Many new city dwellers are poor migrants from rural areas and forced to live in slums in city centres or in the peri-urban areas that surround the city (Brockerhoff and Biddlecom 1999). In Nairobi, slums are affected the most by economic shocks causing a shrinking of the job market in the formal and informal sector; unemployment, which is often the result, has been shown to lead to low school enrolment and pronounced school dropout rates for adolescents (APHRC 2002).

A number of studies in sub-Saharan Africa and Kenya in particular pointed to the link between poverty and sex work among adolescents. This link is also established more generally: Hallman (2004) found that poverty drives sex work among adolescent young women, who are now vulnerable to a higher degree of sexual exploitation and acquisition of HIV and sexually transmitted diseases. According to the Inter-Agency Working Group on Key Populations (2014a), adolescent sex work is very often fuelled by economic disadvantage – 75 per cent of young women aged 12–19 had received money or material goods in exchange for sex in a study conducted in Ghana, Malawi and Uganda. In the town of Kisumu, Kenya, young women reported having received material transfers from male partners in almost 70 per cent of all premarital relationships (Luke et al. 2011). For Robinson and Yeh (2008), the conceptual understanding of the nature of sex-for-money transactions is little understood especially in the context of developing countries in sub-Saharan Africa. Chatterji et al. (2004) based on studies from Cameroon, Kenya, Nigeria, and South Africa found that in many situations, young women exchanged sex for funds to pay education-related expenses as well as a way to provide entry into perceived social networks of influence and power. A technical brief on HIV and young people who sell sex by the Inter-Agency Working Group on Key Populations (2014a) reported that young people sell sex for multiple reasons. These reasons included to escape poverty and meet financial responsibilities such as supporting family when livelihood opportunities are lacking. In Kenya, young sex workers reported having parental responsibilities for their siblings, preferring to sell sex than live in the street (Inter Agency Working Group on Key Populations 2014a). In this regard, a decision was made on 'what was the lesser evil', the course of action of which leads to the least ignominy. Research into survival choices and behaviour preferences is covered to a degree in the literature, but what is lacking is how this relates to a sense of resilience against perceived humiliation and how such action is dignified in the short and long term as 'life-affirming'. Adolescent women in slums have been shown to rely heavily on sex work for meeting basic needs, as subjectively defined and prioritised, such as the desire for consumer items including 'fast food' and 'nice clothing' (Mumah et al. 2014). How these items are ranked and prioritised still needs further explanation in the Nairobi slum as elsewhere.

In South Africa, more than half of street children reported having exchanged sex for money, goods or protection (Inter Agency Working Group on Key Populations 2014a). Economic reasons were identified as the major drivers behind sex work, including homelessness, food insecurity, purchase of clothes, transport as well as procurement of drugs and alcohol. Forced displacement and refugee settings can also increase pressure on young people to exchange sex for material goods or protection. However, the evidence on urban migrant populations and sex work is largely lacking (Inter Agency Working Group on Key Populations 2014a). The Inter-Agency Working Group on Key Populations (2014a) notes that high levels of HIV risk and vulnerability associated with sex work among young people include inconsistent condom use and poor judgement resulting from sustained drug and alcohol use and act as considerable barriers to health care. Young people who sell sex also face legal and policy constraints to reporting abuse. In some cases, formal healthcare settings must report sex work to police. In others, carrying condoms is considered proof of sex work. In their exploration of unintended pregnancies among adolescents in Nairobi slums, Mumah et al. (2014) found that sexual relationships for young people in slums are extremely varied, including same-sex relations, sexual relations with older adults, sex work, romantic relationships with peers, incestuous relationships and multiple concurrent partnerships – all of which put them at risk of contracting HIV to varying degree. Further study in Nigeria in the slums of Ibadan found very high rates of sex work among young people – 29 per cent of male youth and 38 per cent of young women with frequent multiple and concurrent sexual partners and irregular condom use (Adedimeji et al. 2007).

Whereas the causal pathway of poverty and risky sexual behaviour has been well established in the literature, what are less well covered are the multiple definitions, socially constructed, as to what constitutes deprivation and its multiple dimensions. Although Chambers (1995) pointed out that poverty lends itself to diverse interpretation and meanings for different social groups, social status and prestige, family ties and acceptance by the local community are often valued over the more neo-liberalism criteria of wealth through income generation (Chambers 1995). However, this position has rarely informed discussions of urban poverty, humiliation and dignity, and certainly in sub-Saharan Africa. In failing to fully appreciate the complexity of how deprivation and privation are subjectively understood and how they relate to the fear of humiliation, ignominy and ultimately vulnerability, the reasons behind young slum-dwellers' life choices will remain unclear.

Poverty, Gender and Youth

As a critical cross-cutting structural determinant of health, gender[2] is the key factor in understanding disadvantage among the urban poor and provides the lens by which to view overall poorer health status among women (David et al. 2007). Women face multiple vulnerabilities to contracting HIV ranging from biological factors to gender inequality (WHO 2009). Owing to factors of physiology, young women are at heightened risk of HIV infection given the size of the surface area exposed to the virus during sexual intercourse, and HIV infection is more likely in women than men from a single act of unprotected sex (UNAIDS 2004).

---

[2] 'Gender refers to the personal sexual identity of an individual, regardless of the person's biological and outward sex. How people define masculinity and femininity can vary based on the individual's background and surrounding culture. Differing societal expectations in different cultures establish the behavioral, psychological and physical attributes that are associated one gender or another' (Cherry 2015).

In any context, gender inequality creates a situation where young women lack power and autonomy and so have difficulty negotiating HIV prevention practices (Gage 2000). The disempowerment of young women in the sexual sphere and their lack of adequate autonomy to make informed choices and enforce their decisions concerning their sexual lives are critical to discussions on sustaining health (Gage 2000). Autonomy is defined as the degree of women's access to, and control over, finances and material resources; resources, including social status, family and community; and freedom of movement (Bloom et al. 2001). Autonomy in the context of sexual and reproductive health in the literature is very often considered in the context of 'risk' and choice of sexual partners, ability to take affirmative action regarding sexual health and access to fertility and birth facilities (Sen and Batliwala 2000).

It is well noted in the research that at the individual level, many poor women are less able to negotiate safe sexual relations than their male partners, leaving them vulnerable to HIV (Paiva 2000, 2003). According to Tacoli (2012), the unique challenges that young women face in regard to contracting HIV are exacerbated in the urban slum which includes limited control over family resources, responsibilities for child care and tendency towards restricted mobility relative to men.

Evidence from Brazil provides useful illustration. While the country is placed as a leading world economy, it is ranked as 79 on the Human Development Index, a reflection of significant levels of inequality (Agénor and Canuto 2013; UNDP 2014). Pervasive inequality marked by gender, race and social class puts poor women in a very disadvantaged position. HIV trends reflect these inequities (Chacham et al. 2007). In their study of autonomy and susceptibility to HIV among young women living in a Brazilian slum, Chacham et al. (2007) found that indicators of autonomy relating to sexuality, mobility and freedom from threat by partners were significantly correlated with practices linked to HIV prevention and with access to health services promoting prevention.

Young women who were open to discuss condom use with their partner have overall better prevention outcomes. In contrast, those who had ever been a victim of physical violence by a partner or whose partners restricted their mobility were less likely to use condoms (Chacham et al. 2007). The researchers found that information alone related to prevention practices and access to condoms is not enough to assure condom use among adolescents and young women in the informal settlements. While young women knew how to avoid pregnancy and HIV, the question becomes one of autonomy and control over one's own sexuality (Chacham et al. 2007). Studies of Nairobi's slums reveal higher rates of HIV among women for a number of reasons. A study by Hattori and Dodoo (2007) of cohabitation, marriage and sexual monogamy in Nairobi's slums found higher rates of HIV among young females than young males. This was attributed to a number of factors, including that young women have less control over sexual relations, biological factors that make women more susceptible to HIV than men and patterns of sexual networking that contribute to higher infection rates among women. The study also found that women in slum communities in Nairobi have extremely low socioeconomic status, which, for reasons of survival, makes them more likely to report multiple sexual partnerships. In their study of marital status and risk of HIV infection in slum settlements in Nairobi, Kimani-Murage et al. (2013) found that women find it hard to ask their partners to use condoms, even in situations where infidelity is evident. This was due to unfavourable gender power relations and underlying socioeconomic practices, which generally tend to acknowledge that extramarital sex among men is acceptable, but not among women.

Transgender women[3] consistently face heightened vulnerability to HIV. According to a study carried out in 15 countries, transgender women are 49 more times likely to be living with HIV (Inter Agency Working Group on Key Populations 2014b), which sits in stark contrast to other women of reproductive age. Transgender women often gravitate to urban centres where, for reasons not dissimilar to men who have sex with men, the city offers a degree of protection within safe communities and in some cases more liberal attitudes (Baral et al. 2012b). With a limited range of livelihood options owing to overriding social exclusion, urban sex work is often one of the few options for survival. Sex work, practised by any sexual orientation in any place, is high risk for HIV transmission. Faced with hostility and unaccepting health professionals, transgender people often go untreated for sexually transmitted infection, which can, in turn, provide a multitude of risk and vulnerability. As shown by the International HIV/AIDS Alliance (2012), fear of violence or actual violence is often a daily reality for transgender women. In Latin America, 80 per cent of transgender women have experienced violence, typically in the context of urban sex work and from government agents (International HIV/AIDS Alliance 2012). In 2012, the highest number of murders against transgender people and people living with HIV was recorded (Giovanniello 2013). The question of transgender is a little known or researched topic, not just in Kenya but across the continent. The absence is striking given global prevalence rates among transgender women and because it speaks to a silence, born of prejudice, against persons of alternative gender. The global AIDS response, regardless of context, if it is to succeed, must be premised on indivisible human rights (UNAIDS 2011b).

As pointed out by Isiugo-Abanihe (2003), young men have all too often been overlooked in researching sexual and reproductive health of young people. The result is a gap in the evidence concerning their needs, perceptions and motivations in reproductive health matters. This appears to be a crucial gap in sub-Saharan Africa, where males exercise considerable authority in their traditional role of decision-makers both in the home and in society at large (Isiugo-Abanihe 2003). Evidence similarly remains weak concerning the vulnerability of young men who perpetrate sexual violence in sub-Saharan Africa against all people regardless of gender (Ajuwon et al. 2002; Ganju et al. 2004; Jeejebhoy and Bott 2003).

Research carried out in the Caribbean provides further insight into gender power dynamics and notably how risk and vulnerability become socially embedded (Plummer 2009). From this research, a clear gap emerges between knowledge of HIV, which was almost universal, and attitude and practice in regard to risky

---

[3] Transgender is a 'term referring to when one's gender and sex are not always or ever equivalent. Often used as a referent to the person them self. This is a broad term that includes transsexual (pre/ non or post-op), non-gender, bi (tri & multi) gender, androgynists, etc.' (Urban Dictionary 2015).

behaviour. The evident gap between HIV awareness and safe practices among young people is widely known as the 'KAP gap' (knowledge, attitude and practice) and is deeply 'woven into the social fabric' (Plummer 2009, p. 239). This gap countervails social and cultural codes that mitigate against protective behaviour. These socially embedded codes help frame risk and vulnerability. In explaining repeated risk-taking, Plummer (2009) identified five key areas of influence: gender roles, peer group pressures, stigma and taboo, economic power and religion.

For Plummer (2009, 2011), fulfilling male gender roles involved a series of risky obligations. Drawing on a large swathe of research in the Caribbean, the evidence shows that boys are expected to be risk-takers, while, conversely, the expectancy is that girls will be passive (Bailey et al. 1998). Risk-taking, including sexual practices, among boys is culturally engendered. The social expectation to see men and boys as risk-takers is powerful as it is a moral imperative. By contrast, not conforming to mainstream roles and mores, the peer response can be antisocial and even violent (Plummer 2011).

The prevailing expectation is to see 'real males' as 'tough', and a way to pronounce masculine status, especially for younger men, is to have, and be seen to have, multiple female partners. Mensch et al. (2001) stated that young men are subjected to very few hazards but many potential benefits including enhancing social status among peers by engaging in early premarital sex. The cost of not being heterosexually active is to risk social exclusion, ridicule and personal attack (Plummer 2009). Homosexuality is seen as strictly taboo, and homophobia is shown to exercise a profound influence on male risk-taking behaviour that seeks to distance itself, at great cost, from that which could be seen as effeminate (Plummer 2009).

Peer groups play a significant role in the lives of young men. It is within peer groups that masculine codes of conduct are enforced and offer a source for gender norms. Drawing on the work of Chevannes (1999), Plummer (2011) agrees that the peer group has a deep influence on the young male and demands loyalty and respect which is shown through behaviour and attitude. It is within the strictures of the peer group that boys are socialised and learn shared values. Through a process, termed 'rolling peer pressure', peer culture is passed down in multiple settings both formal and informal (Plummer 1999). Much of the messaging concerns sexuality and sexual behaviour considered appropriate is imparted by the peer group which mould male sexual practices. Fulfilment of these expectations will likely enhance standing and status (dignity) of young men among peers regardless of whether it falls out of line with mainstream public health care (Plummer 1999).

Gender roles play a vital component in socially embedding HIV risk; risk is further entrenched by economic power, stigma and religion. Plummer (2011) notes that in certain settings, religion and gender have proved a factor in intensifying HIV risks. These are noted as follows: first, negative messages relating to forms of HIV prevention, notably the use of condoms; second, notions of masculine dominance and engendered sex roles; and, third, through sexual stigma and homophobia which drive the epidemic underground and out of reach.

As part of gender dynamics, money and material assets feature large for defining and protecting male identity. Disposable income means enhanced standing in the group psyche, and acquired wealth could be traded for respect, loyalty and sex (Bailey et al. 1998).

Empirical research that has pointed to poverty as a key driver of the HIV epidemic is arguably too simplistic as it does not take fully into account the entire universe of risk and vulnerability, which cuts across socioeconomic status and location. The epidemic, it has been argued, is being driven by a conflation of both gender norms and money, and risk and vulnerability are shaped by the interrelationship of men, power and wealth. This is further corroborated by studies elsewhere in which HIV prevalence is shown to be markedly higher in locations with concentrations of young men with significant disposable income. This factor has been amply proven in the transport corridors of southern Africa and in the mines of South Africa (Regondi et al. 2013).

References

Abma, J., & McGill, B. (2007, March 29–31). *Teenagers' use of contraceptives at first intercourse: Long-term trends in use, correlates, and predictors for males and females*. Paper presented at the 2007 annual meeting of the Population Association of America. Abstract retrieved from http://paa2007.princeton.edu/papers/71103

Adedimeji, A. A., Omololu, F. O., & Odutolu, O. (2007). HIV risk perception and constraints to protective behaviour among young slum dwellers in Ibadan, Nigeria. *Journal of Health Population and Nutrition, 25*(2). Retrieved from https://www.questia.com/library/journal/1G1-172525512/hiv-risk-perception-and-constraints-to-protective

African Population and Health Research Center. (2002). *Nairobi informal settlements needs assessment survey*. Retrieved from http://www.chs.ubc.ca/archives/files/Health%20and%20Livelihood%20Needs%20of%20Residents%20of%20Informal%20Settlements%20in%20Nairobi%20City.pdf

Agénor, P. R., & Canuto, O. (2013). Gender equality and economic growth: A framework for policy analysis. *VOX Policy Portal*. Retrieved from http://www.voxeu.org/article/gender-equality-and-economic-growth-framework-policy-analysis

Ajuwon, A. J., McFarland, J., Hudes, E. S., Adedapo, S., Okikiolu, T., & Lurie, P. (2002). HIV risk-related behaviour, sexual coercion, and implications for prevention strategies among female apprentice tailors in Ibadan, Nigeria. *AIDS and Behaviour, 6*(3), 229–235. doi:10.1023/A:1019839824312.

Anderson, N., Cockcroft, A., & Shea, B. (2008). Gender-based violence and HIV: Relevance for HIV prevention in hyperendemic countries of southern Africa. *AIDS, 22*(Suppl 4), 73–86. doi:10.1097/01.aids.0000341778.73038.86.

Bailey, W., Branche, C., McGarrity, G., & Stuart, S. (1998). *Family and the quality of gender relations in the Caribbean*. Mona: Institute of Social and Economic Research.

Baral, S., Beyrer, C., Muessig, K., Poteat, T., Wirtz, A. L., Decker, M. R., Sherman, S. G., & Kerrigan, D. (2012a). Burden of HIV among female sex workers in low-income and middle-income countries: A systematic review and meta-analysis. *Lancet Infectious Diseases, 12*(7), 538–549. doi:http://dx.doi.org/10.1016/S1473-3099(12)70066-X.

Baral, S., Poteat, T., Strömdahl, S., Wirtz, A. L., Guadamuz, T. E., & Beyrer, C. (2012b). Worldwide burden of HIV in transgender women: A systematic review and meta-analysis. *Lancet Infectious Diseases, 13*(3), 214–222. doi:http://dx.doi.org/10.1016/S1473-3099(12)70315-8.

Beguy, D., Mumah, J., Wawire, S., Muindi, K., Gottschalk, L., & Kabiru, C. W. (2013). *Status report on the sexual and reproductive health of adolescents living in urban slums in Kenya STEP UP technical working paper*. Nairobi: African Population and Health Research Center.

Bloom, S. S., Wypij, D., & Das Gupta, M. (2001). Dimensions of women's autonomy and the influence on maternal health care utilization in a north Indian city. *Health and Mortality, Demography, 38*(1), 67–78. doi:10.1353/dem.2001.0001.

Brockerhoff, M., & Biddlecom, A. E. (1999). Migration, sexual behaviour and the risk of HIV in Kenya. *International Migration Review, 33*(4), 833–856.

Canadian International Development Agency. (2014). Securing the future of children and youth. *CIDA*. Retrieved from http://www.international.gc.ca/development-developpement/priorities-priorites/cys-sje.aspx?lang=eng

Chacham, A. S., Diniz, S. G., Maia, M. B., Galati, A. F., & Mirim, L. A. (2007). Sexual and reproductive health needs of sex workers: Two feminist projects in Brazil. *Reproductive Health Matters, 15*(29), 108–118. doi:10.1016/S0968-8080(07)29292-4.

Chambers, R. (1995). Poverty and livelihoods: whose reality counts? *Environment and Urbanization, 7*(1), 173–202. Retrieved from http://eau.sagepub.com/content/7/1/173.full.pdf

Chatterji, M., David, N. M., & Anglewicz, L. P. (2004, October). *The factors influencing transactional sex among young men and women in 12 sub-Saharan African countries* (The Policy Project). Retrieved from http://pdf.usaid.gov/pdf_docs/PNADA925.pdf

Cherry, K. (2015). *What is gender?* Retrieved from http://psychology.about.com/od/gindex/g/gender.htm

Chevannes, B. (1999). *What we sow and what we reap – Problems in the cultivation of male identity in Jamaica*. Kingston: Grace Kennedy Foundation.

Cotton, C. (2013). *Research to practice – Strengthening contributions to evidence-based policy making*. Retrieved from https://www.mcqil.ca/isid/files/isid/pd2013otton.pdf

David, A. M., Mercado, S. P., Becker, D., Edmundo, K., & Mugisha, F. (2007). The prevention and control of HIV/AIDS, TB and Vector-borne diseases in informal settlements: Challenges, opportunities and insights. *Journal of Urban Health, 84*(1), 65–74. Retrieved from http://www.ncbi.nlm.nih.gov/pubmed/17431796

Emina, J., Beguy, D., Zulu, E. M., Ezeh, A. C., Muindi, K., Elung'ata, P., Otsola, J. K., & Yé, Y. (2011). Monitoring of health and demographic outcomes in poor urban settlements: Evidence from the Nairobi urban health and demographic surveillance systems. *Journal of Urban Health, 88*(2), 200–218. doi:10.1007/s11524-011-9594-1.

Gage, A. J. (2000). Female empowerment and adolescence: Moving beyond Cairo. In H. Presser & G. Sen (Eds.), *Women's empowerment and demographic processes*. Retrieved from http://econpapers.repec.org/bookchap/oxpobooks/9780198297314.htm

Ganju, D., Jejeebhoy, S., Nidadavolu, V., Santhya, K. G., & Finger, W. (2004). Sexual coercion: Young men's experience as victims and perpetrators. *Popline*. Retrieved from http://www.popline.org/node/267056

Gavin, J. (2000). Arousing suspicion and violating trust: The lived ideology of safe sex talk. *Culture, Health & Sexuality: An International Journal for Research, Intervention and Care*, 117–134. doi:10.1080/136910500300750.

Gibbs, A., Sikweyiya, Y., & Jewkes, R. (2014). 'Men value their dignity': Securing respect and identity construction in urban informal settlements in South Africa. *Global Health Action, 7*. doi:http://dx.doi.org.elibrary.jcu.edu.au/10.3402/gha.v7.23676.

Giovanniello, S. (2013, June 4). *NCAVP report: 2012 hate violence disproportionately target transgender women of color*. Retrieved from http://www.glaad.org/blog/ncavp-report-2012-hate-violence-disproportionately-target-transgender-women-color

Greif, M. J. (2012). Housing, medical, and food deprivation in poor urban contexts: Implications for multiple sexual partnerships and transactional sex in Nairobi's slums. *Health & Place, 18*(2), 400–407. doi:10.1016/j.healthplace.2011.12.008.

Hallman, K. (2004). *Socio economic disadvantage and unsafe sexual behaviours among young women and men in South Africa* (Policy Research Division Working Paper, 190). New York: The Population Council.

Hapern, C. T., & Haydon, A. A. (2012). Sexual timetables for oral-genital, vaginal, and anal intercourse: Sociodemographic comparisons in a nationally representative sample of adolescents. *American Journal of Public Health, 102*(6), 1221–1228. Retrieved from http://search.proquest.com.elibrary.jcu.edu.au/docview/1015208389?pq-origsite=summon

Hattori, M. K., & Dodoo, F. N.-A. (2007). Cohabitation, marriage, and 'sexual monogamy' in Nairobi's slums. *Social Science & Medicine, 64*(5), 1067–1078. doi:10.1016/j. socscimed.2006.10.005.

Inter Agency Working Group on Key Populations. (2014a, July). *HIV and young people who sell sex: A technical brief* (Draft). Retrieved from http://www.who.int/hiv/pub/guidelines/briefs__ sw_2014.pdf?ua=1

Inter Agency Working Group on Key Populations. (2014b, July). *HIV and young transgender people: A technical brief* (Draft). Retrieved from http://www.who.int/hiv/pub/guidelines/ briefs_ykp_2014.pdf?ua=1

International HIV/AIDS Alliance. (2012). *The night is another country: Impunity and violence against transgender women human rights defenders in Latin America.* Retrieved from http:// www.aidsalliance.org/publicationsdetails.aspx?id=90623

Isiugo-Abanihe, U. C. (2003). *Male role and responsibility in fertility and reproductive health in Nigeria.* Retrieved from http://www.worldcat.org/title/male-role-and-responsibility-in-fertility-and-reproductive-health-in-nigeria/oclc/54042707

Jejeebhoy, S. J. & Bott, S. (2003). *Non-consensual sexual experience of young people: A review of the evidence from developing countries* (Working Paper No. 16). Retrieved from http://www. popline.org/node/250871

Joint United Nations Programme on HIV/AIDS (UNAIDS). (2011a). *Place matters HIV in the city.* Unpublished raw data.

Joint United Nations Programme on HIV/AIDS (UNAIDS). (2011b). *A new investment framework for the global HIV response* (UNAIDS Issues Brief). Geneva: UNAIDS.

Joint United Nations Programme on HIV/AIDS (UNAIDS). (2014). *UNAIDS briefing book July 2014.* Geneva: UNAIDS.

Jorgenson, A. K., & Rice, J. (2012). Urban slums and children's health. In F. A. Karides (Ed.) *Journal of World-Systems Research, 18*(1), 103–116. Retrieved from http://www.jwsr.org/wp-content/uploads/2013/02/jorgensonrice-vol18n1.pdf

Juarez, F., & Martin, T. C. (2006). Safe sex versus safe love? Relationship context and condom use among male adolescents in the favelas of Recife, Brazil. *Archives of Sexual Behavior, 35*(1), 25–35. doi:10.1007/s10508-006-8992-z.

Kabiru, C. W., Mojola, S. A., Beguy, D., & Okigbo, C. (2013). Growing up at the margins: Concerns, aspirations and expectations of young people living in Nairobi's slum. *Journal of Research on Adolescence, 23*(1), 81–94. doi:10.1111/j.1532-7795.2012.00797.

Kamndaya, M., Thomas, L., Vearey, J., Sartorius, B., & Kazembe, L. (2014). Material deprivation affects high sexual risk behavior among young people in urban slums, South Africa. *Journal of Urban Health, 91*(3), 581–591. doi:10.1007/s11524-013-9856-1.

Kimani-Murage, E. W., Kyobutungi, C., Ezeh, A. C., Wekesah, F., Wanjohi, M., Muriuki, P., Musoke, R. N., Norris, S. A., Griffiths, P., & Madise, N. J. (2013). Effectiveness of person-alised, home-based nutritional counselling on infant feeding practices, morbidity and nutri-tional outcomes among infants in Nairobi slums: Study protocol for a cluster randomised controlled trial. *Trials, 14*, 445. doi:10.1186/1745-6215-14-445.

Luke, N., Goldberg, R. E., Mberu, B. U., & Zulu, E. M. (2011). Social exchange and sexual behav-ior in young women's premarital relationships in Kenya. *Journal of Marriage & Family, 73*(5), 1048–1064. doi:10.1111/j.1741-3737.2011.00863.x.

Mberu, B. U. (2008). Protection before the harm: The case of condom use at the onset of premarital sexual relationship among youths in Nigeria. *African Population Studies, 23*(1), 57–83. Retrieved from http://www.bioline.org.br/request?ep08004.

Mensch, B. S., Clark, W. H., Lloyd, C. B., & Erulkar, A. S. (2001). Premarital sex, schoolgirl pregnancy and school quality in rural Kenya. *Studies in Family Planning, 32*(4), 285–301. Retrieved from http://www.jstor.org/stable/2696317

Mexico Child Link. (2003). *Street children – What are street children?* Retrieved from http://www. mexico-child-link.org/street-children-definition-statistics.htm

Mugisha, F., Arinaitwe-Mugisha, J., & Hagembe, B. O. N. (2003). Alcohol, substance and drug use among urban slum adolescents in Nairobi, Kenya. *Cities, 20*(4), 231–240. doi:10.1016/ S0264-2751(03)00034-9.

Muindi, K., Mudegeb, N., Beguya, D., & Mberu, B. U. (2014). Migration and sexual behaviour among youth in Nairobi's slum areas. *African Population Studies, 28*(3), 1297–1309.

Mumah, J., Kabriru, C. W., Izugbara, C., & Mukiira, C. (2014, April). *Coping with unintended pregnancies: Narratives from adolescents in Nairobi's slums* (Research Report). Retrieved from www.aphrc.org

Ndola, P., Vahidnia, F., & Fraser, A. (2005). Gender and relationship differences in condom use among 15–24 years old in Angola. *International Family Planning Perspectives, 31*(4), 192–199. Retrieved from http://citeseerx.ist.psu.edu/showciting?cid=18631985

Ngom, P., Magadi, M. A., & Owuor, T. (2003). Parental presence and adolescent reproductive health among the Nairobi urban poor. *Journal of Adolescents Health, 33*(5), 369–377. doi:10.1016/S1054-139X(03)00213-1.

Norr, K., Tlou, S., & Moeti, M. (2004). Impact of peer group education on HIV prevention among women in Botswana. *Health Care for Women International, 25*(3), 210–226. doi:10.1080/07399330490272723.

Paiva, V. (2000). Gendered scripts and the sexual scene. In R. Parker, R. M. Barbosa, & P. Aggleton (Eds.), *Framing the sexual subject: The politics of gender, sexuality and power* (pp. 33–59). Berkeley: University of California Press.

Paiva, V. (2003). Beyond magic solutions: Prevention of HIV/AIDS as a process of psychosocial emancipation. In *Divulgacao para Saude para Debate* (Vol. 27) (pp. 192–203). Retrieved from http://www.saudeemdebate.org.br/

Plummer, D. (1999). *One of the boys; masculinity, homophobia, and modern manhood.* New York: Hawoth Press.

Plummer, D. (2009). How risk and vulnerability become socially embedded: Insights into the resilient gap between awareness and safety in HIV. (Chapter 12). In C. Barrow, M. de Bruin, & R. Carr (Eds.), *Sexuality, social exclusion & human rights: Vulnerability in the caribbean context of HIV* (pp. 239–257). Kingston: Ian Randall Publishing.

Plummer, D. (2011). Masculinity + HIV = Risk: Exploring the relationships between masculinities, education and HIV in the caribbean (chap. 6). In J. F. Klot & V. K. Nguyen (Eds.), *Fourth wave – Violence, gender, culture and HIV in the 21st century* (pp. 139–156). New York: United Nations Educational, Scientific and Cultural Organization.

Regondi, I., George, G., & Pillay, N. (2013). HIV/AIDS in the transport sector of southern Africa: Operational challenges, research gaps and policy recommendations. *Development Southern Africa, 30*(4–05), 616–628. doi:10.1080/0376835X.2013.830239.

Resnick, D., & Casale, C. (2014). Young populations in young democracies: Generational voting behaviour in sub-Saharan Africa. *Democratization, 21*(6), 1172–1194. doi:10.1080/13510347.2013.793673.

Robinson, J., & Yeh, E. (2008). *Transactional sex as a response to risk in western Kenya* (MPRA_paper_7405). Retrieved from http://mpra.ub.uni-muenchen.de/7405/

Sen, G., & Batliwala, S. (2000). Empowering women reproductive rights. In H. B. Presser & G. Sen (Eds.), *Women's empowerment and demographic processes: Moving beyond Cairo* (pp. 15–36). Oxford: Oxford University Press.

Shafil, T., Stovel, K., Davis, R., & Holmes, K. (2004). Is condom use habit forming? Condom use at sexual debut and subsequent condom use. *Sexually Transmitted Diseases, 31*(6), 366–372. doi:10.1097/00007435-200406000-00010.

Tacoli, C. (2012). Urbanization, gender and urban poverty: paid work and unpaid carework in the city. International Institute for Environment and Development & United Nations Population Fund. Urbanization and Emerging Populations Issues, Working Pater 7. Retrieved from http://pubs.iied.org/10614IIED.html.

Tumwesigye, N. M., Ingham, R., & Holmws, D. (2005, April). *Condom use at first and most recent sex among unmarried people aged 15–24 in Uganda: A case of Kabala and Mukono Districts.* Paper presented at the seminar organized by the University of Southampton, Centre for AIDS Research (CAR), UK. Abstract received from http://slideplayer.com/slide/4511404/

United Nations Children's Fund (UNICEF). (2010). *Progress for children – Achieving the MDGs with equity* (No. 9). New York: UNICEF.

United Nations Children's Fund (UNICEF). (2012). *State of the world's children. Children in an urban world.* Retrieved from http://www.unicef.org/sowc2012/

United Nations Children's Fund (UNICEF) & Joint United Nations Programme on HIV/AIDS (UNAIDS). (2004). *The framework for the protection, care and support of orphans and vulnerable children living with HIV/AIDS.* New York: UNICEF.

United Nations Development Programme (UNDP). (2014). *Sustaining human progress: Reducing vulnerabilities and building resilience. Human development report 2014.* Retrieved from http://hdr.undp.org/en/content/human-development-report-2014

United Nations Human Settlements Programme (UN–Habitat). (2013a). *State of urban youth report 2012/2013. Youth in the prosperity of cities.* Retrieved from http://issuu.com/unhabitatyouthunit/docs/state_of_the_urban_yourh_report_201

United Nations Human Settlements Programme (UN–Habitat). (2013b). *Streets as public spaces and drivers of urban prosperity.* Retrieved from http://unhabitat.org/books/streets-as-public-spaces-and-drivers-of-urban-prosperity/

United Nations Human Settlements Programme (UN–Habitat). (2014a, April 5–11). *World urban forum, urban equity in development – Cities for life.* Medellin. Retrieved from https://www.facebook.com/worldurbanforum

United Nations Human Settlements Programme (UN–Habitat). (2014b, May 14). *Harnessing the dual global trends of urbanization and the demographic youth bulge* (Issues Paper). Retrieved from http://www.un.org/en/ecosoc/julyhls/pdf13/hls_issue_note_un_habitat.pdf

United Nations Human Settlements Programme (UN–Habitat). (2014c). *CEB high-level committee on programmes. Twenty-seventh session.* Retrieved from http://unhabitat.org/

Urban Dictionary. (2015). *Transgender.* Retrieved from http://www.urbandictionary.com/define,php?term=transgender&defid=546786

William, K. A., & Alexander, C. S. (1999). Determinants of condom use to prevent HIV infection among youth in Ghana. *Journal of Adolescent Health, 24,* 63–72. doi:10.1016/S1054-139X(98)00062-7.

World Bank. (2015a). *East Asia's changing urban landscape: Measuring a decade of spiritual growth.* Retrieved from http://www.worldbank.org/en/topic/urbandevelopment/publication/east-asias-changing-urban-landscape-measuring-a-decade-of-spatial-growth

World Bank. (2015b). *OVC toolkit.* Retrieved from http://info.worldbank.org/etools/docs/library/162495/howknow/definitions.htm

World Health Organisation (WHO). (2009). *Women and health: Today's evidence, tomorrow's agenda.* Retrieved from http://www.who.int/gender-equity-rights/en/

Chapter 5
Migration, Young People and Vulnerability in the Urban Slum

Abstract This chapter examines the universe of risk and resilience and focuses on sexual and reproductive health among the growing number of young migrants taking up residence in the urban slum.

Keywords HIV • Urban slums • Young people • Urban migrants • Internally displaced people • Urban refugees • Mobile populations • Sexual and reproductive health • Social capital • Dignity and humiliation • Kenya

Migrants and Mobile Populations

According to Zimmerman et al. (2011), population mobility has now become a defining policy issue. Major drivers of this mobility are economic, sociocultural, sociopolitical and environmental as well as inter- and intra-state conflict (Zimmerman et al. 2011). For developing countries, migration is often an adaptive social response to climate change (UNISDR 2014) leading to the idea of 'climate refugees'. Increasingly scarce resources in rural areas and the promise of economic opportunity in urban areas contribute to a rise in urban migration – and the growth of informal settlements (UN-Habitat 2012). Migration, especially in search for economic opportunity, is central to understanding the HIV dynamic in Africa, as it is elsewhere. This is well documented in southern Africa. As Lurie (2006) showed, migrants working in the South African mines exposed to social and economic vulnerabilities can engage in risky sexual behaviour, notably through the possession of disposable income. As a consequence, research must now prioritise a disaggregated analysis of HIV vulnerability, risk and resilience relevant to all forms of migrancy (International Organization on Migration and African Population and Health Research Center 2015) and highlight the major aspects of that vulnerability and resilience.

Drawing on a multi-country analysis, UN-Habitat (2007a) shows that Nairobi is one of the fastest growing cities in Africa. The city's exponential growth illustrates a rapid urbanisation along with a mushrooming of city slums (UN-Habitat 2007a). The population of Nairobi has increased tenfold since the 1960s mostly as a result of natural increment and rural to urban migration (APHRC 2014). A significant but largely unknown number are urban migrants, which includes asylum seekers and migrant workers in regular or irregular situations constantly arriving into the city.[1] At the start of 2014, there was an estimated half a million refugees and over 52,000 asylum seekers throughout Kenya (United Nations High Commissioner for Refugees (UNHCR) 2014). In 2011, some 46,000 refugees and 11,000 asylum seekers were residing in Nairobi (UNHCR 2011). Campbell et al. (2011) have shown that given obstacles in collating strategic information, urban migrancy into Nairobi remains something of an unknown. From their work, a best guess is that the number of migrant workers approximates 80,000–100,000 (Campbell et al. 2011). Campbell et al. (2011) agree with earlier findings that all types of migrants are widely dispersed mainly throughout informal settlements across Nairobi (Dix 2006; Pavanello et al. 2010).

Migration and Sexual and Reproductive Health

While migration is not in itself a risk factor for poor health, conditions surrounding the migration process for the vast part increase vulnerabilities to ill health and HIV. Migrant adolescents and youth with irregular status studied in urban areas and along transit routes in and around cities have been shown to face barriers in accessing basic services, owing to factors of higher fees compared to nationals, cultural and language barriers, low health literacy including knowledge of the health system, real or perceived hostility by health-care workers and host community members and the absence of caregivers for young people (IOM 2011b). Migrants subjected to exclusion, alienation and anonymity and in particular migrants in an irregular situation can be disproportionately vulnerable to contracting disease and developing mental health problems (IOM 2011b). Those parts of the city with concentrations of migrants are often difficult to reach with health information and services, and HIV programmes, already overstretched with the burden of disease in host communities, are not structured to cater for the needs of 'invisible' populations such as refugees, asylum seekers and undocumented migrants (IOM 2011b).

A wide body of literature shows that across all continents, migration is associated with riskier behaviour, including sexual risk behaviour (Baumer and South 2004; Brockerhoff and Biddlecom 1999; Greif and Dodoo 2011; Sambisa and Stokes 2006; IOM 2011a). Sampson and Laub (1993) in the early 1990s found that migration from rural to urban centres is often associated with the weakening of existing bonds, which can in turn lead to an increased likelihood of nontraditional behaviours. Beck et al. (1991) found that social control factors, such as religious systems,

---

[1] The broad classifications for migrancy are economic migrant, documented/regular migrant, irregular/non-documented migrant, refugee and asylum seeker.

socioeconomic position and family ties, affect the strength of these bonds in diverse ways during and after migration, a situation still evidenced today. Despite this early finding, research has not arguably sufficiently explored the matter of migration and social bonds including mobility to and from the slums of Nairobi. The disruption of social networks can lead to patterns of nonnormative behaviour and give way to feelings of isolation and dislocation among migrants, factors shown to be key in understanding humiliation and risky behaviour (South et al. 2005). Young migrants, in particular, tend to gain easier acceptance into peer groups with higher rates of deviance including violent crime (Haynie et al. 2006; South et al. 2005).

Brockerhoff and Biddlecom (1999) provided a framework for studying differences in overall behaviour of migrants, based on three broad lines of analysis: predisposing individual characteristics, changes in individual attributes due to migration, notably separation from a spouse or partner and exposure to a new social environment, with different sexual norms, opportunities and constraints that hold an influence over sexual behaviour. These three perspectives have over the course of the past two decades helped explain fertility differences between migrants and non-migrants as well as further explained the selectivity of migration, life disruptions associated with mobility and migrants' adaptation to social expectations in new places of residence.

Mberu and White (2011) review the 'selectivity hypothesis', which posits that migrants are not randomly selected, but migration is selective in regard to personal characteristics such as higher education, young age, unmarried status and desire for upward social mobility. Attributes of these migrants predispose their behaviour to be different from nonmigrants, particularly regarding risky sex. According to the authors, the disruption hypothesis in the period immediately following migration is associated with physiological stress due to moving, loss of social capital and separation from significant others. The 'adaptation hypothesis' proposes that migrants adapt to the new economic, social and cultural environment at the places of destination, often resulting in marked behaviour change (Mberu and White 2011). The very act of making this voluntary movement, which often takes place over distance and time and between different sociocultural environments, with uncertain outcomes helps define migrants as inherent risk-takers (Mberu 2008, citing Peterson 1958; Massey et al. 1994). Moreover, migrants from the outset may be predisposed towards heightened risk-taking behaviour, including engaging in risky sex (Mberu 2008, citing Brockerhoff and Biddlecom 1999). Risk-taking patterns of voluntary and non-voluntary migrants to the urban slums and particularly regarding patterns of convergence and assimilation need further investigation, especially given that both forms of migrancy to urban centres are increasing, globally.

The global evidence reflects these arguments. Residential change, from one known universe to another, is associated with increased premarital and extramarital sexual relationships (Halli et al. 2007; Mberu and White 2011). These behaviours are all strongly associated with transmission of HIV and sexually transmitted disease (STD) (Lurie 2006). Research into urban contexts in sub-Saharan Africa has documented that poor sexual and reproductive outcomes are shaped by early sexual debut, a factor often associated with migration (Gage 1998; Gregson et al. 2005;

Harrison et al. 2005; Pettifor et al. 2004). Drawing on data from the 2008 Nigeria Demographic and Health Survey, one study examined the patterns of internal migration and sexual initiation among never-married Nigerian youth aged 15–24 and showed that migrants generally demonstrate stronger association than nonmigrants and urban to rural and rural to rural migrants in particular, with premarital sexual initiation (Mberu and White 2011). In their study of the migration experience and premarital sexual initiation in urban Kenya, Luke et al. (2012) found that young people, both male and female, who migrate, either alone or as a family unit, during early adolescence tend to engage more in sexual activity. Luke et al. (2012) also pointed to the link between changes in place of residence with multiple and concurrent sexual partners, premarital and extramarital sexual relationships and inconsistent condom use. Migration into urban areas, as held, exposes individuals to new ideas, more permissive social norms and sexual networks. Luke et al. (2012) conclude that migration during formative adolescence and early adult years often leads to early sexual debut and other unsafe sexual practices.

The literature shows that the situation of adolescent young women is complex. Certain dimensions of migration offer a degree of protection against early sexual initiation based on the number of residential changes in the last 1–3 months (Mberu and White 2011). Another study looking at youth in urban Kenya found that young women who migrated in the past month were two times more likely to enter a second (concurrent) sexual partnership, compared with those who did not recently migrate (Xu et al. 2010). The interaction between migration and behaviour change is complex and context dependent (Smith 1999). The literature also demonstrates that in Africa migration very often takes place within family and community networks and is a valuable form of support in helping young people adjust to life in a new environment. These ties affect the sexual behaviour of young migrants, especially adolescent young women. Adolescent young women often face additional restrictive norms than boys and greater parental and community control of their behaviour, which has offered a degree of protection against risky sex (Browing et al. 2005; Luke et al. 2011b).

Age of migration is a critical factor in understanding vulnerability and resilience (Luke et al. 2012). It is posited that early adolescents will face greater adjustment difficulties than they would at later ages, particularly when they are less resilient to change (Luke et al. 2012). Lacking cognitive maturity, as Dixon-Mueller (2008) shows, young adolescents, particularly boys, can be driven to engage in risk-taking and sensation-seeking behaviour, including sexual activity. Young women, however, may be more vulnerable to disruptions caused by migration during early adolescence owing to emotional and physical changes associated primarily with puberty and residential change and effect a 'downward assimilation' to peer groups identified with risky behaviour (Luke et al. 2012). The evidence suggests that young women who faced early disruption but do not experience subsequent moves is an important factor in determining vulnerability and risky sexual behaviour (Luke et al. 2012). However, despite the evident differences in developmental and social processes between adolescent boys and young women, there is a noted lack of research on gender and sexual activities in the context of migration and in particular intra-urban mobility.

Harrison et al. 2005; Pettifor et al. 2004). Drawing on data from the 2008 Nigeria Demographic and Health Survey, one study examined the patterns of internal migration and sexual initiation among never-married Nigerian youth aged 15–24 and showed that migrants generally demonstrate stronger association than nonmigrants and urban to rural and rural to rural migrants in particular, with premarital sexual initiation (Mberu and White 2011). In their study of the migration experience and premarital sexual initiation in urban Kenya, Luke et al. (2012) found that young people, both male and female, who migrate, either alone or as a family unit, during early adolescence tend to engage more in sexual activity. Luke et al. (2012) also pointed to the link between changes in place of residence with multiple and concurrent sexual partners, premarital and extramarital sexual relationships and inconsistent condom use. Migration into urban areas, as held, exposes individuals to new ideas, more permissive social norms and sexual networks. Luke et al. (2012) conclude that migration during formative adolescence and early adult years often leads to early sexual debut and other unsafe sexual practices.

The literature shows that the situation of adolescent young women is complex. Certain dimensions of migration offer a degree of protection against early sexual initiation based on the number of residential changes in the last 1–3 months (Mberu and White 2011). Another study looking at youth in urban Kenya found that young women who migrated in the past month were two times more likely to enter a second (concurrent) sexual partnership, compared with those who did not recently migrate (Xu et al. 2010). The interaction between migration and behaviour change is complex and context dependent (Smith 1999). The literature also demonstrates that in Africa migration very often takes place within family and community networks and is a valuable form of support in helping young people adjust to life in a new environment. These ties affect the sexual behaviour of young migrants, especially adolescent young women. Adolescent young women often face additional restrictive norms than boys and greater parental and community control of their behaviour, which has offered a degree of protection against risky sex (Browing et al. 2005; Luke et al. 2011b).

Age of migration is a critical factor in understanding vulnerability and resilience (Luke et al. 2012). It is posited that early adolescents will face greater adjustment difficulties than they would at later ages, particularly when they are less resilient to change (Luke et al. 2012). Lacking cognitive maturity, as Dixon-Mueller (2008) shows, young adolescents, particularly boys, can be driven to engage in risk-taking and sensation-seeking behaviour, including sexual activity. Young women, however, may be more vulnerable to disruptions caused by migration during early adolescence owing to emotional and physical changes associated primarily with puberty and residential change and effect a 'downward assimilation' to peer groups identified with risky behaviour (Luke et al. 2012). The evidence suggests that young women who faced early disruption but do not experience subsequent moves is an important factor in determining vulnerability and risky sexual behaviour (Luke et al. 2012). However, despite the evident differences in developmental and social processes between adolescent boys and young women, there is a noted lack of research on gender and sexual activities in the context of migration and in particular intra-urban mobility.

socioeconomic position and family ties, affect the strength of these bonds in diverse ways during and after migration, a situation still evidenced today. Despite this early finding, research has not arguably sufficiently explored the matter of migration and social bonds including mobility to and from the slums of Nairobi. The disruption of social networks can lead to patterns of nonnormative behaviour and give way to feelings of isolation and dislocation among migrants, factors shown to be key in understanding humiliation and risky behaviour (South et al. 2005). Young migrants, in particular, tend to gain easier acceptance into peer groups with higher rates of deviance including violent crime (Haynie et al. 2006; South et al. 2005).

Brockerhoff and Biddlecom (1999) provided a framework for studying differences in overall behaviour of migrants, based on three broad lines of analysis: predisposing individual characteristics, changes in individual attributes due to migration, notably separation from a spouse or partner and exposure to a new social environment, with different sexual norms, opportunities and constraints that hold an influence over sexual behaviour. These three perspectives have over the course of the past two decades helped explain fertility differences between migrants and nonmigrants as well as further explained the selectivity of migration, life disruptions associated with mobility and migrants' adaptation to social expectations in new places of residence.

Mberu and White (2011) review the 'selectivity hypothesis', which posits that migrants are not randomly selected, but migration is selective in regard to personal characteristics such as higher education, young age, unmarried status and desire for upward social mobility. Attributes of these migrants predispose their behaviour to be different from nonmigrants, particularly regarding risky sex. According to the authors, the disruption hypothesis in the period immediately following migration is associated with physiological stress due to moving, loss of social capital and separation from significant others. The 'adaptation hypothesis' proposes that migrants adapt to the new economic, social and cultural environment at the places of destination, often resulting in marked behaviour change (Mberu and White 2011). The very act of making this voluntary movement, which often takes place over distance and time and between different sociocultural environments, with uncertain outcomes helps define migrants as inherent risk-takers (Mberu 2008, citing Peterson 1958; Massey et al. 1994). Moreover, migrants from the outset may be predisposed towards heightened risk-taking behaviour, including engaging in risky sex (Mberu 2008, citing Brockerhoff and Biddlecom 1999). Risk-taking patterns of voluntary and non-voluntary migrants to the urban slums and particularly regarding patterns of convergence and assimilation need further investigation, especially given that both forms of migrancy to urban centres are increasing, globally.

The global evidence reflects these arguments. Residential change, from one known universe to another, is associated with increased premarital and extramarital sexual relationships (Halli et al. 2007; Mberu and White 2011). These behaviours are all strongly associated with transmission of HIV and sexually transmitted disease (STD) (Lurie 2006). Research into urban contexts in sub-Saharan Africa has documented that poor sexual and reproductive outcomes are shaped by early sexual debut, a factor often associated with migration (Gage 1998; Gregson et al. 2005;

Luke et al. (2012) discuss migration and assimilation which involves numerous processes that serve to shape young people's sexual behaviour. The key to patterns of assimilation is socioeconomic integration into new locations, which in turn impacts health behaviours including mortality and nutritional status (Luke et al. 2012, citing Akresh 2007; Venters and Gany 2011; Reed et al. 2012). A large body of evidence points to the fact that migrants' health often deteriorates over time in the new location including increasingly engaging in unsafe sexual activities (Luke et al. 2012). Furthermore, adolescents and young adults experiencing a new normative environment can feel traumatised and isolated in their efforts to integrate into peer networks (Luke et al. 2012). The notion of family disruption through change of residence especially for already traumatised young people may well add to the sense of loss and substantially challenges resilience at all levels (Hosegood et al. 2007; Madhavan 2004; Mberu 2008). Empirical research has so far not explored if those experiences that can lead to humiliation for the young migrant are significantly different from the mobile intra-slum resident. Short of pointing to the wide practice of transactional sex as a means of survival, measures available to each social group to significantly 'dignify' their respective worlds remain unclear.

The evidence indicates that residential change and family disruption during adolescence and early adulthood can have an effect on long-term health and developmental behaviours (South et al. 2005). Finding themselves in an alien environment, young people, as part of their efforts to assimilate, may seek out peer groups that encourage early sexual activity (South et al. 2005). Earlier research from North America indicates that the number of residential moves impact young people's sexual behaviour as with each move, the likelihood of premarital sex increased by a factor of 5 per cent among 15–19-year-olds, which is reflected in the experience drawn from related findings in Nairobi (Stacks 1994). One conclusion drawn from this research is that numerous residential moves create a sense of transiency that gives way to temporary casual relationships. Again, the literature still fails to explain the long-term impact on sexual choices for migrants' once long-term residency has been established and notably in highly insecure environments.

Women migrants, in particular, can face heightened vulnerability to HIV. Reasons given are vulnerability to sexual abuse and violence, neglect for their reproductive health needs and marginalisation from education, employment, goods and services (Carballo et al. 1996). In a study of HIV transmission and acquisition risk among female migrants in Kenya, Camlin et al. (2014) found that gendered aspects of the migration process – the circumstances that trigger migration, livelihood strategies available to female migrants and social features of migration destinations – are often associated with high risks of contracting HIV. Migrations were often triggered within the household often due to changes in marital status and gender-based violence (Camlin et al. 2014). The evidence also showed that female migrants are often forced to engage in sex work as a way of supplementing earnings from informal sector trading. Additional evidence from Kenya indicates that young female urban migrants in Kenya often turn to sex work to earn a living and generally lack access to reproductive health services and crucial information and support for HIV prevention and treatment (Ngugi et al. 2012; IOM 2011a). Despite the fact that the Kenyan national response is increasingly targeting research and programming towards key population groups, migrant female sex workers are not seen as a discreet group. IOM (2011a) reported that in one study carried out among migrant female sex workers in Nairobi, half (52.2 per cent) were between the ages of 20 and 29 and with an overall HIV prevalence of 23.1 per cent. The study also demonstrated low levels of education and literacy among migrant female sex workers, making it harder to find work in the formal employment sector; and whereas nearly all respondents had heard of HIV, knowledge around prevention and transmission was mixed and demonstrated with many misconceptions (IOM 2011a). The report concluded that migrant female sex workers are marginalised by social determinants of health, in particular, irregular migration status, lack of fluency in local languages and cultural barriers (IOM 2011a).

Migrant Health in the Urban Slum

Though the links are well established, less work has been carried out to investigate the sexual and reproductive health of migrants, particularly young migrants, in the urban slums of sub-Saharan Africa. A few studies look at the health of child migrants more broadly in the urban slums. Bocquier et al. (2011) note that children of migrating parents born and living in Nairobi's congested informal settlements have a higher mortality rate than non-slum-born children. Children born in the slums to women who were pregnant at the time of migration have the highest risk of dying (Bocquier et al. 2011).

Greif and Dodoo (2011) note that in Kenya, rural to urban migration is central to the high levels of urbanisation and to the growth of slum settlements, with Nairobi's slums being now the home to a majority of the city's population (Zulu et al. 2002). Migratory factors, specifically previous place of residence and length of time spent in the urban slum since arrival, are all important in shaping the outcome of migrants' health. Zulu et al. (2002) found a connection between the likelihood of engaging in risky sex in urban settings and the area of origin for migrants. However, what needs further explanation is how behaviour patterns change in urban settings as a result of social media, school, home and formal health settings. Such study would shed light on the nexus of vulnerability as well as the pressure points concerning risk, ill health, vulnerability and resilience.

Refugees and Internally Displaced People in Kenya

In Kenya, as elsewhere, there is ample evidence to show that refugees often experience trauma as a result of conflict and displacement (Onyut et al. 2009). In trying to reassert normality to their lives, refugees find opportunities in accessing income or resources severely challenging, a factor directly relating to vulnerability to national response is increasingly targeting research and programming towards key population groups, migrant female sex workers are not seen as a discreet group. IOM (2011a) reported that in one study carried out among migrant female sex workers in Nairobi, half (52.2 per cent) were between the ages of 20 and 29 and with an overall HIV prevalence of 23.1 per cent. The study also demonstrated low levels of education and literacy among migrant female sex workers, making it harder to find work in the formal employment sector; and whereas nearly all respondents had heard of HIV, knowledge around prevention and transmission was mixed and demonstrated with many misconceptions (IOM 2011a). The report concluded that migrant female sex workers are marginalised by social determinants of health, in particular, irregular migration status, lack of fluency in local languages and cultural barriers (IOM 2011a).

Migrant Health in the Urban Slum

Though the links are well established, less work has been carried out to investigate the sexual and reproductive health of migrants, particularly young migrants, in the urban slums of sub-Saharan Africa. A few studies look at the health of child migrants more broadly in the urban slums. Bocquier et al. (2011) note that children of migrating parents born and living in Nairobi's congested informal settlements have a higher mortality rate than non-slum-born children. Children born in the slums to women who were pregnant at the time of migration have the highest risk of dying (Bocquier et al. 2011).

Greif and Dodoo (2011) note that in Kenya, rural to urban migration is central to the high levels of urbanisation and to the growth of slum settlements, with Nairobi's slums being now the home to a majority of the city's population (Zulu et al. 2002). Migratory factors, specifically previous place of residence and length of time spent in the urban slum since arrival, are all important in shaping the outcome of migrants' health. Zulu et al. (2002) found a connection between the likelihood of engaging in risky sex in urban settings and the area of origin for migrants. However, what needs further explanation is how behaviour patterns change in urban settings as a result of social media, school, home and formal health settings. Such study would shed light on the nexus of vulnerability as well as the pressure points concerning risk, ill health, vulnerability and resilience.

Refugees and Internally Displaced People in Kenya

In Kenya, as elsewhere, there is ample evidence to show that refugees often experience trauma as a result of conflict and displacement (Onyut et al. 2009). In trying to reassert normality to their lives, refugees find opportunities in accessing income or resources severely challenging, a factor directly relating to vulnerability to

Luke et al. (2012) discuss migration and assimilation which involves numerous processes that serve to shape young people's sexual behaviour. The key to patterns of assimilation is socioeconomic integration into new locations, which in turn impacts health behaviours including mortality and nutritional status (Luke et al. 2012, citing Akresh 2007; Venters and Gany 2011; Reed et al. 2012). A large body of evidence points to the fact that migrants' health often deteriorates over time in the new location including increasingly engaging in unsafe sexual activities (Luke et al. 2012). Furthermore, adolescents and young adults experiencing a new normative environment can feel traumatised and isolated in their efforts to integrate into peer networks (Luke et al. 2012). The notion of family disruption through change of residence especially for already traumatised young people may well add to the sense of loss and substantially challenges resilience at all levels (Hosegood et al. 2007; Madhavan 2004; Mberu 2008). Empirical research has so far not explored if those experiences that can lead to humiliation for the young migrant are significantly different from the mobile intra-slum resident. Short of pointing to the wide practice of transactional sex as a means of survival, measures available to each social group to significantly 'dignify' their respective worlds remain unclear.

The evidence indicates that residential change and family disruption during adolescence and early adulthood can have an effect on long-term health and developmental behaviours (South et al. 2005). Finding themselves in an alien environment, young people, as part of their efforts to assimilate, may seek out peer groups that encourage early sexual activity (South et al. 2005). Earlier research from North America indicates that the number of residential moves impact young people's sexual behaviour as with each move, the likelihood of premarital sex increased by a factor of 5 per cent among 15–19-year-olds, which is reflected in the experience drawn from related findings in Nairobi (Stacks 1994). One conclusion drawn from this research is that numerous residential moves create a sense of transiency that gives way to temporary casual relationships. Again, the literature still fails to explain the long-term impact on sexual choices for migrants' once long-term residency has been established and notably in highly insecure environments.

Women migrants, in particular, can face heightened vulnerability to HIV. Reasons given are vulnerability to sexual abuse and violence, neglect for their reproductive health needs and marginalisation from education, employment, goods and services (Carballo et al. 1996). In a study of HIV transmission and acquisition risk among female migrants in Kenya, Camlin et al. (2014) found that gendered aspects of the migration process – the circumstances that trigger migration, livelihood strategies available to female migrants and social features of migration destinations – are often associated with high risks of contracting HIV. Migrations were often triggered within the household often due to changes in marital status and gender-based violence (Camlin et al. 2014). The evidence also showed that female migrants are often forced to engage in sex work as a way of supplementing earnings from informal sector trading. Additional evidence from Kenya indicates that young female urban migrants in Kenya often turn to sex work to earn a living and generally lack access to reproductive health services and crucial information and support for HIV prevention and treatment (Ngugi et al. 2012; IOM 2011a). Despite the fact that the Kenyan

HIV. From an HIV Behavioural Surveillance Survey report (Intergovernmental Authority on Development and United Nations High Commissioner on Refugees (UNHCR) (2010)) carried out in Dadaab Refugee Camp in Kenya, home to more than a quarter million refugees, poverty, displacement and food insecurity were all shown to greatly increase vulnerability to contracting HIV (IGAD and UNHCR 2010). Mobility of refugees is associated with accentuated levels of high-risk sexual behaviour, including casual and transactional sex. Highly mobile refugees, in particular young women, are more likely to have experienced forced sex (IGAD and UNHCR 2010). As the authors of the report state, longer trips outside the camp increase the chances of sexual interaction with other populations having a higher prevalence of HIV. Whereas the subject of forced sex is often underreported, 9 per cent of women and 3 per cent of men still reported experiences of forced sex (IGAD and UNHCR 2010). In another study, IOM (2011b) notes that the constant movement of refugees between countries of origin, refugee camps and urban centres like Nairobi creates the means of introducing and transmitting communicable disease, including HIV. Further study elaborating on these initial findings has proved difficult owing to laws of internal refugee movement and especially concerning urban settings in Kenya.

It is reckoned that approximately two-thirds of the world's forcibly uprooted people are displaced within their own country (UNHCR 2012). This population group are the 'internally displaced people' (IDP).[2] At the end of 2012, there was an estimated 28.8 million IDP around the world, a substantial increase from 2011 (UNHCR 2012). At the end of 2013, there were more than 51 million people worldwide who had been forcibly displaced, the highest number since the end of the Second World War (UNAIDS 2015b). Sub-Saharan Africa is the region with the largest number of IDPs, estimated at 10.4 million, an increase of 7.5 per cent compared with 2013 (UNHCR 2015b). Forced dislocation is a key contributing factor of HIV and consistent vulnerability.

Arguably the largest group of vulnerable people in the world, urban IDPs are often denied with basic human rights, are forced to live in sub-human conditions and lack physical security and freedom of movement (Fielden 2008). Unrecognised and undocumented by their government, they often lack sufficient food, water, health care, education and livelihoods (Fielden 2008). Women and children displaced in urban areas are documented as being especially vulnerable to sexual and gender-based violence (Fielden 2008). Furthermore, the experience of poor sanitation has been documented as being detrimental to the reproductive health of urban IDP women (Fielden 2008). Disempowered IDP women, in particular, suffer for the lack of income-generating activities (Fielden 2008).

Available evidence indicates that an increasing number of people have been uprooted and forced to seek solace away from traditional and rural homes in Kenya. Tens of thousands of households in Kenya have been internally displaced in recent years – an estimated 300,000 in 1992, 150,000 in 1997, 20,000 in 2002 and, most

---

[2] An internally displaced person is someone who is forced to flee his or her home but who remains within his or her country's borders (UNHCR 2015b).

recently, 660,000 in 2007/2008 as a result of postelection violence (Kamungi 2013). Eight districts in Nairobi were recorded as having high population densities of IDP, in particular, Central Nairobi (49 per cent), Kasarani (43 per cent) and Embakasi (40 per cent) (Norwegian Refugee Council (NRC) and Internal Displacement Monitoring Centre (IDMC) 2011). The IDMC (2013) reported there were an estimated 412,000 IDP in Kenya at the start of 2014. Reasons given for the experience of displacement in Kenya are intercommunal conflict, politically instigated violence, issues surrounding land tenure and the increasing occurrence of rapid-onset disaster. The target zones for these IDP are mostly Mandera, Wajir, Lamu, Turkana and Nairobi (Kamungi 2013; OCHA 2015).

Major periods of violence and displacement in Kenya centred on the 1992 and 1997 general elections (NRC and IDMC 2011). In 2007, allegations of election irregularities and malpractice led to widespread violence and thousands of displaced persons. The violence disproportionately affected communities living in Nairobi slums, notably Kibera, Gatwikira, Bombolulu, Soweto, Kiandaa, Mashimoni and Mathare where youths allied with opposing political parties clashed, resulting in significant loss of life and property (NRC and IDMC 2011). The result was widescale movement of impoverished populations across the country's informal slum settlements. These areas have continued to be most affected by recurrent urban displacement (Kamungi 2013).

Following the 2007 violence, people displaced in Nairobi took refuge in pockets across the city. By 2008, more than 30 official and unofficial IDP sites were documented in and around Nairobi (Kamungi 2013). For many, the so-called durable solution has never been a reality.[3] Once settled and integrated, IDP are no longer eligible for forms of external (government) support having fulfilled the requirements of the 'integrated solution' (NRC and IDMC 2011).

Landless and in many cases separated from family members, IDP found and continue to do so their way into slum settlements seeking any form of employment and sustenance (NRC and IDMC 2011). Kamungi (2013) described the business environment in the urban slum following the 2007/2008 postelection violence as unpredictable owing to violence and other shocks. Furthermore, this report detailed violence in the Nairobi urban slums as severely disrupting all forms of livelihoods including established trading networks. Survival mechanisms adopted by some IDP households included the forced separation of children and dependents from primary caregivers to other locations causing trauma among those responsible for these children and for the children themselves (Kamungi 2013). A longitudinal study of these young displaced persons which seeks to draw out the exact nature of vulnerability and risk and empowerment has as yet to be conclusively carried out.

---

[3] International law defines three 'durable solutions' for refugees: voluntary repatriation, local integration and resettlement (Azad and Jasmin 2013). A 'durable solution' is when IDP are not considered as having any specific assistance and protection needs directly relating to their displacement and as such enjoy their human rights without discrimination on account of their displacement (Kamungi 2013).

Njiru (2014) states that owing in part to congestion and lack of privacy in over-crowded households hosting IDP, incidents of violence and abuse are not uncommon including numerous cases of reported child labour and sexual exploitation. The complexity and scope of vulnerability of orphans and displaced children to urban areas and especially for adolescent girls has been documented (Birdthistle et al. 2008). The Kenya Human Rights Commission (KHRC) (2009) observed that in Eldoret town, following the violence of 2007/2008, hundreds of school-aged children turned to urban begging as a means of survival. However, the value system of begging, scavenging and dignity in the urban slum requires much further study and one that is able to depict the social universe of a subculture often alien to the researcher.

As shown in a profiling study of migrants' and nonmigrants' vulnerability in Nairobi, the continuing flow of IDP to Nairobi is a sign that life is becoming harder to sustain in rural areas and other smaller urban centres (NRC and IDMC 2011). Whereas this study showed the differences between IDP and economic migrants' experiences in Nairobi as unremarkable, there was a substantial difference compared with nonmigrants owing primarily to nonmigrants' level of social capital (NRC and IDMC 2011). The report demonstrated that IDP are more likely to live in high-risk areas, less likely to own their own dwelling and have larger households, including more children (NRC and IDMC 2011). The report also found that IDP tend to be younger than other migrants and that both IDP and migrants had lower levels of education than nonmigrants with women much less likely to hold a higher education degree than men (NRC and IDMC 2011).

IDP arriving in Kenya's cities are a consequence of involuntary migration and very often arrive with particular needs and few, if any, material assets with which to build new lives. As is the case with many other mobile populations, IDP must start life afresh in what may be an alien and unfamiliar environment (IOM 2011a, c). The evidence shows that IDP often share a dwelling with other households and are more likely than other groups to live in a shack settlement with less rooms and to share these rooms with more people and to live in unsafe areas such as landslide-prone areas, garbage mountains, railroads or industrial areas (NRC and IDMC 2011). IDP are less securely employed than other groups and more likely to work part-time, experience higher rates of crime and physical attack and are less likely to know about or participate in local community organisations (NRC and IDMC 2011). The evidence is wanting regarding the matter of IDP social cohesion, and what does exist has tended to focus on questions of integration and assimilation and less so on quality of life defined on their terms.

Many IDP seek refuge in urban and peri-urban areas with extended family networks or members of the same ethnic communities (Inter Agency Standing Committee 1993). In Kenya, involuntary migration has occurred in waves usually as a result of a downward turn in rural homes. However, as the IDMC (2014) states as each new wave arrives, the effect is a further burdening on the preceding wave of displaced people who are now expected to provide a measure of support and assistance for the new arrivals. The long-term result is a further impoverishment of the IDP family unit (IDMC 2014; Kamungi 2013). Nyawira (2014) reports that IDP living in Nairobi slums do not enjoy their full gamut of human rights, lacking protection, access to social services and security of tenure. Vulnerability needs therefore to be understood in terms of time, assimilation and diminishing resources. The impact of shrinking options and livelihood choices on dignity and humiliation, vulnerability and resilience is wholly absent from the literature.

There remain gaps in the critical information on Kenya's urban IDP. Previous municipal authorities in Kenya did not, as a rule, collect demographic data on migration patterns into urban centres. The problem is further exacerbated by the question of 'integrated IDP' and how they can be singled out from the population of humanitarian concern with whom they now reside (Fielden 2008; Nyawira 2014). Making distinctions between resident and IDP vulnerability has often been shown to be a spurious exercise given overriding levels of humanitarian need inclusive of shelter, food and accessible health services faced by all slum inhabitants.

References

African Population and Health Research Center. (2014). *Population and health dynamics in Nairobi's informal settlements. Report of the Nairobi Cross-sectional Slums Survey (NCSS) 2012*. Nairobi: African Population and Health Research Center.

Akresh, I. R. (2007). Dietary assimilation and health among Hispanic immigrants to United States. *Journal of Health and Social Behavior, 48*(4), 404–417. doi:10.1177/002214650704800405.

Azad, A., & Jasmin, F. (2013). Durable solutions to the protracted refugee situation: The case of Rohingyas in Bangladesh. *Journal of Indian Research, 1*(4), 25–35, ISSN: 2321–4155.

Baumer, E. P., & South, S. J. (2004). Community effects on youth sexual activity. *Journal of Marriage and Family, 63*(2), 540–554. doi:10.1111/j.1741-3737.2001.00540.x.

Beck, S. C., Cole, B. S., & Hammond, J. A. (1991). Religious heritage and premarital sex. *Journal of the Scientific Study of Religion, 30*(2), 173–180. doi:10.2307/1387211.

Birdthistle, I., Floyd, S., Machingura, A., Mudziwapasi, N., Gregson, S., & Glynn, J. R. (2008). From affected to infected? Orphanhood and HIV risk among female adolescents in urban Zimbabwe. *AIDS, 22*(6), 759–766. doi:10.1097/QAD.0b013e3282f4cac7.

Bocquier, P., Beguy, D., Zulu, E. M., Muindi, K., Konseiga, K., & Ye, Y. (2011). Do migrant children face greater health hazards in slum settlements? Evidence from Nairobi, Kenya. *Journal of Urban Health, 88*(2), 266–281. doi:http://dx.doi.org/10.1007%2Fs11524-010-9497-6.

Brockerhoff, M., & Biddlecom, A. E. (1999). Migration, sexual behaviour and the risk of HIV in Kenya. *International Migration Review, 33*(4), 833–856.

Browing, R. B., Leventhal, T., & Brooks-Gunn, J. (2005). Sexual initiation in early adolescence: The nexus of parental and community control. *American Sociological Review, 70*(5), 758–778. Retrieved from http://asr.sagepub.com/content/70/5/758.abstract

Camlin, C. S., Kwena, Z. A., & Dworkin, S. L. (2014). "She mixes her business": HIV transmission and acquisition risks among female migrants in western Kenya. *Social Science & Medicine, 102*(February 2014), 146–156. doi:10.1016/j.socscimed.2013.11.004.

Campbell, E., Crisp, J., & Kiragu, E. (2011). *Navigating Nairobi: A review of the implementation of UNHCR's urban refugee policy in Kenya's capital city*. Geneva: UNHCR.

Carballo, M., Grocutt, M., & Hadzihasanovic, A. (1996). Women and migration: A public health issue. *World Health Quarterly, 49*(2), 158–164.

Dix, S. (2006). Urbanization and the social protection of refugees in Nairobi. *Humanitarian Exchange Magazine, 35*. Retrieved from http://www.odihpn.org/humanitarian-exchange-magazine/issue-35/urbanisation-and-the-social-protection-of-refugees-in-nairobi

Dixon-Mueller, R. (2008). How young is 'too young'? Comparative perspectives on adolescents sexual, marital and reproductive transition. *Studies in Family Planning, 39*(4), 247–262. Retrieved from http://www.jstor.org/stable/20454474

Fielden, A. (2008). *Ignored displaced person: The plight of IDPs in urban areas. New issues in Refugee Research* (Research Paper No. 161). Retrieved from http://www.refworld.org/docid/4c2325690.html

Gage, A. J. (1998). Sexual activity and contraceptive use: The component of the decision making process. *Studies in Family Planning, 29*(2), 154–166. Retrieved from http://www.jstor.org/discover/10.2307/172156?uid=3738336&uid=2&uid=4&sid=21106634278193

Gregson, S., Nyamukapa, C. A., Garnett, G. P., Wambe, M., Lewis, J. J. C., Mason, P. R., Chandiwana, S. K., & Anderson, R. M. (2005). HIV infection and reproductive health in teenage women orphaned and made vulnerable by AIDS in Zimbabwe. *AIDS Care: Psychological and Socio-medical Aspects of AIDS/HIV, 17*(7), 785–794. doi:10.1080/09540120500258029.

Greif, M. J., & Dodoo, F. (2011). Internal migration to Nairobi's slums: Linking migration streams to sexual risk behavior. *Health & Place, 17*, 86–93.

Halli, S. S., Blanchard, J., Satihal, D. G., & Moses, S. (2007). Migration and HIV transmission in rural South India: An ethnographic study. *Culture, Health and Sexuality, 9*(1), 85–94. Retrieved from http://www.ncbi.nlm.nih.gov/pubmed/17364716

Harrison, A., Cleland, J., Gouws, E., & Frohlich, J. (2005). Early sexual debut among young men in rural South Africa: Heightened vulnerability to sexual risk? *Sexual Transmitted Infections, 81*(3), 259–261. doi:10.1136/sti.2004.011486.

Haynie, D. L., South, S. J., & Bose, S. (2006). The company you keep: Adolescent mobility and peer behavior. *Sociological Inquiry, 76*(3), 397–426. doi:10.1111/j.1475-682X.2006.00161.x.

Hosegood, V., Floyd, S., Marston, M., Hill, C., McGrath, N., Isingo, R., Crampin, A., & Zab, B. (2007). The effects of high HIV prevalence on orphanhood and living arrangements of children in Malawi, Tanzania, and South Africa. *Population Studies, 61*(3), 327–336. Retrieved from http://www.ncbi.nlm.nih.gov/pubmed/17979006

Inter Agency Standing Committee. (1993). *Internally displaced persons outside camps: Achieving a more equitable humanitarian response.* New York: United Nations.

Intergovernmental Authority on Development & United Nations High Commissioner on Refugees (UNHCR). (2010). *HIV behavioural surveillance survey in Dadaab refugee camps.* Geneva: UNHCR.

Internal Displacement Monitoring Centre. (2013). *Kenya IDP figures analysis.* Retrieved from http://www.internal-displacement.org/sub-saharan-africa/kenya/figures-analysis

Internal Displacement Monitoring Centre & the Norwegian Refugee Council. (2014). *Too early to turn the page on IDPs, more work in needed.* Retrieved from www.internal-displacement.org

International Organization on Migration and African Population and Health Research Center (2015). Regional synthesis on patterns and determinants of migrants' health and associated vulnerabilities in urban setting of East and Southern Africa. Johannesburg: International Organization on Migration

International Organization for Migration (IOM). (2011a). *Integrated biological and behavioural surveillance survey among migrant female sex workers in Nairobi, Kenya 2010. Healthy migrants in healthy communities.* Retrieved from the International Organization for Migration website: http://health.iom.int/

International Organization for Migration (IOM). (2011b). *An analysis of migration health in Kenya – Healthy migrants in healthy communities.* Retrieved from the International Organization for Migration website: http://health.iom.int/

International Organization for Migration (IOM). (2011c). *IOM, glossary on migration* (International Migration Law Series No. 25). Retrieved from https://www.iom.int/key-migration-terms.

Joint United Nations Programme on HIV/AIDS (UNAIDS). (2015a). *The critical role of communities in reaching global targets to end the AIDS epidemic.* Retrieved from the Relief Web website: http://reliefweb.int/report/world/communities-deliver-critical-role-communities-reaching-global-targets-end-aids-epidemic

Joint United Nations Programme on HIV/AIDS (UNAIDS). (2015b). *HIV and humanitarian emergencies.* Retrieved from http://safaids.net/content/hiv-and-humanitarian-emergencies

Joint United Nations Programme on HIV/AIDS (UNAIDS). (2015c). UNAIDS regional support team for Eastern and Southern Africa. Retrieved from http://www.unaidsrsstesa.org/region/region-profile

Joint United Nations Programme on HIV/AIDS (UNAIDS). (2015d, February 17). All in to end adolescent AIDS. *Reliefweb*. Retrieved from http://reliefweb.int/report/world/all-endadolescentaids

Kamungi, P. (2013). *Municipalities and IDPs outside of camps: The case of Kenya's 'integrated' displaced persons*. Retrieved from http://reliefweb.int/report/kenya/municipalities-and-idps-outside-camps-case-kenya%E2%80%99s-%E2%80%98integrated%E2%80%99-displaced-persons

Kenya Human Rights Commission. (2009). *Out in the cold: The fate of internally displaced persons in Kenya 2008–2009*. Retrieved from www.khrc.or.ke

Luke, N., Clark, S., & Zulu, E. M. (2011a). The relationship history calendar: Improving the scope and quality of data on youth sexual behavior. *Demography, 48*(3), 1151–1176. doi:10.1007/s13524-011-0051-2.

Luke, N., Goldberg, R. E., Mberu, B. U., & Zulu, E. M. (2011b). Social exchange and sexual behavior in young women's premarital relationships in Kenya. *Journal of Marriage & Family, 73*(5), 1048–1064. doi:10.1111/j.1741-3737.2011.00863.x.

Luke, N., Xu, H., Mberu, B. U., & Goldberg, R. E. (2012). Migration experience and premarital sexual initiation in urban Kenya: An event history analysis. *Studies in Family Planning, 43*(2), 115–126. Retrieved from http://www.ncbi.nlm.nih.gov/pmc/articles/PMC3665273/

Lurie, M. N. (2006). The epidemiology of migration and HIV/AIDS in South Africa. *Journal of Ethnic and Migration Studies, 32*(4), 649–666. doi:10.1080/13691830600610056.

Madhavan, S. (2004). Fosterage patterns in the age of AIDS: Continuity and change. *Social Science and Medicine, 58*(7), 1443–1454. Retrieved from http://www.ncbi.nlm.nih.gov/pubmed/14759688

Massey, D. S., Gross, A. B., & Shibuya, K. (1994). Migration, segregation, and the geographic concentration of poverty. *American Sociological Review, 59*(3), 425–445. Retrieved from http://www.jstor.org/stable/2095942

Mberu, B. U. (2008). Protection before the harm: The case of condom use at the onset of premarital sexual relationship among youths in Nigeria. *African Population Studies, 23*(1), 57–83. Retrieved from http://www.bioline.org.br/request?ep08004.

Mberu, B. U., & White, M. J. (2011). Internal migration and health: Premarital sexual initiation in Nigeria. *Social Science and Medicine, 72*(8), 1284–1293. doi:10.1016/j.socscimed.2011.02.019.

Ngugi, E., Benoit, C., Hallgrimsdottir, H., Jansson, M., & Roth, E. A. (2012). Partners and clients of female sex workers in an informal urban settlement in Nairobi, Kenya. *Culture, Health & Sexuality: An International Journal for Research, Intervention and Care, 14*(1), 17–30. doi:10.1080/13691058.2011.608436.

Njiru, R. (2014). Political battles on women's bodies: post-election conflicts and violence against women in internally displaced persons camps in kenya. Societies without borders 9(1), 48–68. Retrieved from https://societieswithoutborders.files.wordpress.com/2014/04/njiru-final.pdf.

Norwegian Refugee Council & Internal Displacement Monitoring Centre. (2011, December). *IDP profiling survey in Nairobi*. Retrieved from http://www.bing.com/search?q=).+IDP+Profiling+survey+in+Nairobi.&src=IE-SearchBox&FORM=IENTTR&conversationid=

Nyawira, L. (2014, November 25). IDPs accuse Kenyan Government of ignoring them. *Standard Digital*. Retrieved from http://www.sde.co.ke/m/

Onyut, L. P., Neuner, F., Ertl, V., Schauer, E., Odenwald, M., & Elbert, T. (2009). Trauma, poverty and mental health among Somali and Rwandese refugees living in an African refugee settlement – An epidemiological study. *Conflict Health, 3*(6). doi:10.1186/1752-1505-3-6.

Pavanello, S., Elhawary, S., & Pantuliano, S. (2010). *Hidden and exposed: Urban refugees in Nairobi, Kenya* (HPG Working Paper). Retrieved from HPG website: www.odi.org.uk/sites/odi.org.uk/files/odi-assets/publications-opinion-files/5858.pdf

Peterson, W. (1958). A general typology of migration. *American Sociological Review, 23*(3), 256–266. Retrieved from http://www.jstor.org/stable/2089239

Pettifor, A. E., Straten, A. V. D., Megan, S. D., Shiboski, S. C., & Padian, S. N. (2004). Early age at first sex: A risk factor for HIV infection among women in Zimbabwe. *AIDS, 18*(10),

1435–1442. Retrieved from http://journals.lww.com/aidsonline/Fulltext/2004/07020/Early_age_of_first_sex___a_risk_factor_for_HIV.10.aspx

Reed, H. E., Catherine, S. A., Luke, N., & Fuentes, L. (2012, May 3–5). *The health of African immigrants in the U.S.: Explaining the immigrant health advantages.* Poster presented at the annual meeting of the Population Association of America, San Francisco. Abstract retrieved from http://paa2012.princeton.edu/papers/121968

Sambisa, W., & Stokes, C. S. (2006). Rural/urban residence, migration, HIV/AIDS, and safe sex practices among men in Zimbabwe. *Rural Sociology, 71*(2), 183–211. doi:10.1526/003601106777789684.

Sampson, R., & Laub, J. (1993). *Crime in the making.* Cambridge: Harvard University Press.

Smith, D. J. (1999). *Having people: Fertility, family and modernity in Igbo speaking Nigeria* (Doctoral dissertation, Emory University, Department of Anthropology, Atlanta). Retrieved from http://www.africabib.org/rec.php?RID=W00095481&DB=w

South, S. J., Haynie, D. L., & South, S. B. (2005). Residential mobility and the onset of adolescent sexual activity. *Journal of Marriage and Family, 67*(2), 499–514. Retrieved from http://www.jstor.org/stable/3600284

Stacks, S. (1994). The effect of geographic mobility on premarital sex. *Journal of Marriage and Family, 56*(1), 204–208.

United Nations High Commissioner for Refugees (UNHCR). (2011). *Global trends 2010.* Retrieved from http://www.unhcr.org/4dfa11499.htlm

United Nations High Commissioner for Refugees (UNHCR). (2012). Internally displaced people, on the run in their own land. Retrieved from http://www.unhcr.org/pages/49c3646c146.html

United Nations High Commissioner for Refugees (UNHCR). (2014). *Update on the impact of the Government directive and security operation Usalama watch on refugees and asylum-seekers in urban areas of Kenya.* Retrieved from http://mhpss.net/resource/update-on-the-impact-of-the-government-directive-and-security-operation-usalama-watch-on-refugees-and-asylum-seekers-in-urban-areas-of-kenya/

United Nations High Commissioner for Refugees (UNHCR). (2015a). *Refugee and Asylum seekers in Kenya, 2015.* Retrieved from http://reliefweb.int/report/kenya/refugees-and-asylum-seekers-kenya-mar-15

United Nations High Commissioner for Refugees (UNHCR). (2015b). *Refugees by numbers.* Retrieved from http://www.unhcr.org/pages/49c3646c23.html

United Nations High Commissioner for Refugees (UNHCR). (2015c). *UNHCR country operations profile-Kenya. Overview.* Retrieved from http://www.unhcr.org/pages/49e483a16.html

United Nations Human Settlements Programme (UN–Habitat). (2007a). *Kenya slum upgrading project.* Strategy Document. Retrieved from http://nairobiplanninginnovations.com/projects/kenya-slum-upgrading-programme-kensup/

United Nations Human Settlements Programme (UN–Habitat). (2007b). *Enhancing urban safety and security. Global report on human settlements.* Retrieved from http://unhabitat.org/

United Nations Human Settlements Programme (UN–Habitat). (2012). *Contribution of UN-Habitat to the annual MDG report.* Retrieved from http://unhabitat.org/

United Nations Office for Disaster Risk Reduction (UNISDR). (2014) *Urban risk reduction and resilience.* Retrieved from www.unisdr.org

United Nations Office for the Coordination of Humanitarian Affairs (UN/OCHA). (2015). *Kenya humanitarian overview.* Retrieved from https://fts.unocha.org/pageloader.aspx?page=emerg-emergencyCountryDetails&cc=ken

Venters, H., & Gany, F. (2011). African immigrant health. *Journal of Immigrant Minority Health, 13*(2), 333–344. doi:10.1007/s10903-009-9243-x.

Xu, H., Luke, N., & Zulu, E. (2010). Concurrent sexual partnerships among youth in urban Kenya: Prevalence and partnership effects. *Population Studies, 64*(3), 247–261. doi:10.1080/00324728.2010.507872.

Zimmerman, C., Kiss, L., & Hossain, M. (2011). Migration and health: A framework for 21st century policy-making. *PLoS Medicine.* doi:10.1371/journal.pmed.1001034. Published: 2011, May 24.

Zulu, E., Dodoo, F. N.-A., & Ezeh, A. C. (2002). Sexual risk-taking in the slums of Nairobi, Kenya, 1993–98. *Population Studies: A Journal of Demography, 56*(3), 311–323. doi:10.1080/00324720215933.

Chapter 6
Discussion and Conclusion

Abstract This chapter provides a discussion of the major findings and conclusions drawn from the literature review. Learnings from the research suggest that to end AIDS, the study of dignity and humiliation and especially in the context of young people's vulnerability, risk and resilience to HIV must form part of the emerging urban strategy.

Keywords Ending AIDS • Young people • Dignity and humiliation • Vulnerability • Risk • Resilience • Urban slums • Gender • Urban research

The 'normal professionalism' informed by neo-liberalism that has dominated research into poverty-related vulnerability relevant to the urban slum pointed to by Chambers (1995) still needs rethinking and reformulating. In the light of continuing socioeconomic change and associated migration patterns, conventional frames of reference and tools of investigation must be critically reviewed in both rural and urban settings (Smith and King 2011). The HIV epidemic continues apace in the informal slum settlement and in itself points to weaknesses in the established approach towards and definition of vulnerability, deprivation and urban survival. Empirical enquiry to date has rarely tackled the complexity of resilience and dignity and its practical underpinnings concerning risky behaviour and HIV. What are wholly missing in the literature are recent studies that aim to depict the social universe of young people, be they migrant or multigenerational resident, and how they themselves construct an understanding of the concepts of vulnerability, risk and resilience.

Research into urban environments can quickly appear outdated, even irrelevant, concerning the drivers of HIV vulnerability. Urban spaces are expanding and patterns of urban life changing. Cities, especially in Africa, are becoming younger. Ending AIDS, globally, is being increasingly seen in the context of asserted and informed action carried out in the cities of sub-Saharan Africa. Research, however, is being challenged to keep up with current urban developments and particularly regarding young people and associated patterns of risk and behaviour. The exponential growth of unplanned and uncoordinated urban spaces has its most complete

G. Jones, *HIV and Young People: Risk and Resilience in the Urban Slum*,
SpringerBriefs in Public Health, DOI 10.1007/978-3-319-26814-9_6

expression in the informal slum settlement that has tested conventional notions of the 'urban dynamic' and left wholly wanting accepted understandings of what constitutes urban prosperity and advantage. In the light of these changes, conventional understanding of the plight of urban slum inhabitants must now be critically examined alongside the need to reformulate a better suited paradigm of research and analysis which adequately captures the energy and perception of the subjects of research.

Evidence shows that young people in African urban environments engage in increased sexual activity, yet current knowledge remains inconclusive regarding the complexity and inter-relational nature of likely underlying causes. What has been highlighted as factors of vulnerability is the role of delayed age of marriage, universal education, falling age of puberty, omnipresence of Western mass media and entertainment, notions of individualism and erosion of traditional values and social control (Mberu 2012; National Research Council and Institute of Medicine 2005). Yet the interplay of these factors has been little explored, and given changes in perception and ranking of priorities among young people, much of the evidence has more historical than current value. Cross-sectional research has rarely dealt with the diversity of life and livelihood and associated status currencies in the urban slum. Following a review of the literature, there is a compelling need to study – from the point of view of young slum-dwellers – their perception of change, status and how to escape the reach of vulnerability and want including their very real attempts to dignify a life lived in a slum. Moreover, such research must consider the evident contradictions in knowledge, attitude and practice and the role of subculture value systems that make sense of the world and define acceptable and non-acceptable behaviour. The normal professionalism needs to know much more about young slum-dwelling population's needs, preferences and priorities within the social sphere (Mberu 2012).

Vulnerability and humiliation as experienced by young people differ according to place, time, age and maturity, a determining factor but one which is often absent from a wide body of literature. There must be an in-depth insight into the subjective interpretation of vulnerability and resilience and notably in the context of sexual and reproductive health of young people (Mberu et al. 2014). More so, how this resilience relates to notions of dignifying an existence lived in a climate of violence and uncertainty is yet to be established by empirical fact. The temporal dimension of youth remains overlooked, notably the profound difference between younger and older adolescents and their respective perception of risk, safety and security, especially for migrants living in an alien environment.

This review has shown that in agreement with Mberu et al. (2014), the evidence pertaining to young people's sexual and reproductive health remains incomplete. Scholarly enquiry must add to the knowledge concerning key populations and young people most at risk to HIV infection, which needs to include unemployed young men searching for identity within the limits of the unregulated informal sector (Amaziga 1997; Arowujolu et al. 2002; Slap et al. 2003). Studies carried out in Nairobi have shown that both young men and women in certain situations shy away from formal health care and go unnoticed from population-based survey instruments. They thus become hidden populations. Yet without access to formal health care for these groups, the goal of ending AIDS is untenable. Mainstream research on vulnerability and wellbeing which has tended to look to the provision and uptake of formal health services by 'hetero-normal' men and women as the benchmark creates gaps in the evidence regarding other key populations.

Men have routinely been overlooked in research on young people and particularly so in matters relating to sexual and reproductive behaviour. The result is a substantial gap in the evidence regarding needs, perceptions and motivations of young men and its impact on the choices available for young women. As depicted by Isiugo-Abanihe (2003), within the overriding African patriarchal context in which males exercise authority in their traditional role of decision makers, failing to understand young men's behaviour and sexuality continues to present a major gap in the evidence. Research has shown a commonality of perception by young men and women towards key aspects of vulnerability, but differences emerge regarding questions of resilience, sexual violence and sexual coercion. What is known is that young men and women will likely experience humiliation in different ways and seek alternative solutions all of which have a profound effect on health and wellbeing.

Gender and vulnerability, including research into HIV, have largely taken a binary approach: male or female. The question of vulnerability of same sex liaisons while much discussed for males and to a lesser extent females, however, has bypassed other forms of gender and remains strikingly absent in the literature on vulnerability in urban centres. The literature neglects to take into account the interaction within and between different gender groups and the impact this holds on perceptions of health, dignity and resilience.

Demographic and ethnographic data on urban settings, as a rule, needs to go much further in unravelling the profound differences between slum, intra-slum and non-slum settlement necessary for unpacking the social construct of risk and resilience. Survival for many young people living in the urban slum necessitates a constant movement within and between physical locations and social groups, yet the evidence remains inconclusive regarding its impact on the critical factors of risk and humiliation. The subjective perception of risk, resilience and social status held by young people living and transiting within different slum locations categorised along lines of vulnerability and deprivation needs to be fully understood and noted in the context of HIV and vulnerability. Questions of social, distal and proximal mobility within the context of slum life have yet to be fully explored and especially in the light of increasing numbers of new arrivals into the evolving urban space. Accordingly, research on intra-urban vulnerability to HIV must further develop the appropriate tools and indicators to fully understand the dynamic and complex nature of mobility and social mixing relevant to the different age cohorts of young people.

The literature demonstrates heterogeneity as a major feature in describing slum and non-slum areas of the city. Research carried out in the informal settlements of Nairobi has shown marked differences in patterns of vulnerability between subpopulations including urban refugees, internally displaced persons, economic migrants and multigenerational slum-dwellers. Drawing on theories of social capital, the place of social currencies and how they are understood and utilised from the point of view of young slum-dwelling people as well as their role in 'hedonistic adaptation' to promote standing and status within the local community requires comprehensive explanation through informed qualitative ethnographic enquiry. Similarly, the point of convergence in behaviour patterns between young migrants and resident remains poorly understood, as does the formulation and outcomes of perceptions of humiliation and personal and collective strength.

In Kenya, the 'populations of humanitarian concern' are growing many of whom reside or frequently travel to Kenya's urban slums. Understanding the complexity of vulnerability and the options for a resilient dignity relevant for these populations and the impact of their assimilation into mainstream urban life is still, as the literature suggests, in its infancy. Given the increasing numbers involved in rural to urban migration, and particularly involuntary migration, that many of these groups head to places of inherent instability and structural deprivation, contextualised research needs now to further explore the inter-relational effect on humiliation and vulnerability between the slum populations and what this holds for HIV prevention, treatment and care.

The structural constraints and inherent instability of the slum are invariably explained in terms of poverty and deprivation. That said, how notions of deprivation affect the many dimensions of vulnerability, powerlessness and humiliation has yet to be established by empathetic research nor has research to date comprehensively identified the 'how to' measure a dignified resilience among slum-dwelling populations, especially for young people. Although the connection between per capita GDP and wellbeing is well noted in the literature, the constructs of humiliation, shame, self-respect and social status, also seen as components of health-seeking behaviour, are not easily measured by empirical tools and consequently go largely unmeasured and undetected.

A growing body of evidence has made the connection between forced dislocation of the migrant and humiliation and its impact on compounding the scope and depth of vulnerability (Hartling 2005). What is now required is research into the effect of dislocation, humiliation, attitude and behaviour in the context of urban slum life for these migrant populations. For such research, Nairobi and cities in eastern and southern Africa provide a fertile ground as for many commentators it is 'the perfect storm' of risk and vulnerability.

In a quickly changing physical environment, much more needs to be known about the impact, or more precisely, the complexity of HIV infection in slums in Kenya, as is the case for other cities in sub-Saharan Africa. The gap in the evidence is striking given that HIV remains a major cause of mortality and morbidity among the urban poor. Yet the impact of HIV is still arguably under-researched for the urban poor in Kenya even though an estimated 70 % of all urban dwellers in Nairobi live in one form of slum or 'shack settlement' (UN-Habitiat 2006). What is known is that slum residents are more adversely affected by the HIV epidemic than non-slum counterparts and exhibit the worse health indicators in the country (Ross and Mirowsky 2011).

There are still gaps in the evidence regarding uptake of the tools of HIV prevention, including condom use. Directly relevant to the question of risk and resilience among sexually active young people, the evidence base is weak owing to an over-reliance on standard survey tools testing 'knowledge, attitudes and correct and consistent use of condoms' and not the intricate relationship between the immedi-ate environment involving culture and religion and messaging on sexual and repro-ductive behaviour for African youth (Bankole et al. 2007). How condom use serves to dignify sexual relations and/or how 'unsafe sex' may be felt preferable given the immediate rewards it brings which directly impact upon health and wellbeing requires further research.

In Kenya, as in other sub-Saharan countries, the question of urban migration and sexual activity and young people is an emerging field of research. What enquiry has been conducted (Luke et al. 2012) has prioritised quantitative analysis in the exami-nation of migration and sexual behaviour. It is reported that sex work often consti-tutes an important livelihood activity for migrant women, yet the intersection of mobile populations and 'risky sex' is relatively underexplored (Richter et al. 2014). Similarly significant is the lack of research on gender and sexual activities in the context of migration especially noting the evident differences in developmental and social processes between adolescent boys and girls (Luke et al. 2012). Published data on the prevalence of risky sex as displaced populations settle into urban slums in postemergency settings, across the board, needs strengthening (Spiegel et al. 2014). There is a clear need for fresh insights into the nature of risk among migrant populations and especially young migrants' sexual behaviour during the process of maturation (Platt et al. 2013).

For unravelling the complexity of vulnerability, risk and resilience, the literature shows an absence of high-quality empirical evidence. The time is right for a qualita-tive research that enquires more into the nature of vulnerability, HIV and health outcomes which compliments well-crafted quantitative study. Such research should take note of the apparent disconnect between methodological positions as well as research techniques demonstrated in context-specific settings premised on well-known theories about vulnerability, risk and resilience. What is called for is research that helps shape a theoretical framework for the ecological and multilevel relation-ships among young people in the urban slum as they relate to HIV infection and wellbeing. Population-based surveys much used as the empirical evidence for fur-ther study in Kenya have not provided the depth of evidence critical for understand-ing the nuances of individual perception of vulnerability and resilience among migrant and nonmigrant communities.

The major gap that needs to be addressed is the lack of focus on perception, sta-tus, knowledge and resilience of young people and in creating a sense of self and identity within the structural determinants of the slum and, ultimately, how this impacts on behaviour and prevention of HIV. Enquiry of this nature needs to build on existing research and provide further insight into the pressing issue of health care for young migrant and nonmigrant populations living in hitherto unrecognised parts of the city (Ngware et al. 2013), that is, research which explores how young men and women discover and apply knowledge of HIV and make sense of their vulnerability underpinned by the need for social acceptance, social status and socio-economic gain. In drawing on previous work, such research would examine notions of social currency (Samson 2014) and 'trade-offs' in health-seeking behaviour to achieve a greater perceived personal goal. Young people seek to dignify their lives and livelihoods and do so using a set of references or significant life events often intelligible to them alone. Research needs to identify if the act of dignifying life and livelihood by young people from different social groups is a major factor in preventing or spreading HIV.

The reality for urban-dwelling poor in modern African cities has not been captured in a way that emphasises the 'local and specific' that gives justice to its complexity and diversity and reflects the largely experimental approach to life of its inhabitants in achieving a sense of wellbeing. A research project that seeks to address this gap and presents the case from the point of view of these same slum residents is critical. In so doing, an account can be made of the multiple realities that exist and the multidimensional nature of deprivation itself. Short of a wholly unexpected development in the trajectory of the epidemic, slum-dwelling residents in Nairobi, as across Africa, shall continue to bear the brunt of HIV (Kyobutungi et al. 2008). Given the complexity of researching 'risky' sexual behaviour and particularly in the slum environment, further scholarly work is called for to generate much needed information that provides a holistic picture of the totality of vulnerability for young people all of whom are infected and affected to varying degrees by HIV and AIDS.

UNAIDS believes that there now exists a real window of opportunity to break the global HIV epidemic (UNAIDS 2014a). Accordingly, seeing urban centres as key to ending AIDS, UNAIDS has called for a 'fast-track city response'. If concerted and well-informed measures are taken between 2015 and 2020, the evidence holds that the epidemic can be controlled leading to its eventual demise by 2030 when it no longer represents a public health threat. It is estimated that ending the AIDS epidemic by 2030 would save 21 million lives and that, globally, 28 million new HIV infections and 21 million AIDS-related deaths will be inverted between now and 2030 (UNAIDS 2014b). Conversely, if these efforts fail, then the HIV trajectory will likely again rise and on a greater scale than before. As part of the fast-track initiative, the evidence must be strengthened in diverse ways and generate information in less explored areas particularly regarding the interpersonal nature of vulnerability, dignity and resilience. A review of the literature leads to the conclusion that to end AIDS, there must be more innovative research on the matter of subjective interpretation of health and wellbeing that shapes the universe of young slum-dwelling populations. At the heart of this work is to understand the effect of perceived or actual humiliation and the myriad ways taken by young people in the urban slum to establish a life that is resilient as it is dignified.

References

Amaziga, U. S. (1997). Sexual activity and contraceptive knowledge and use among in- school adolescents in Nigeria. *International Family Planning Perspectives, 23*(1), 28–33.

Arowujolu, A. O., Ilesanmi, A. O., Roberts, O. A., & Okunola, M. A. (2002). Sexuality, contraceptive choice, and AIDS awareness among Nigeria undergraduates. *African Journal of Reproductive Health, 6*, 60–70.

Bankole, A., Ahmed, F. H., Neema, S., Ouedraogo, C., & Konyani, S. (2007). Knowledge of correct condom use and consistency of use among adolescents in four countries in sub-Saharan Africa. *African Journal of Reproductive Health, 11*(3), 197–220.

Chambers, R. (1995). Poverty and livelihoods: whose reality counts? *Environment and Urbanization, 7*(1), 173–202. Retrieved from http://eau.sagepub.com/content/7/1/173.full.pdf

Hartling, L. (2005). *Humiliation: Real pain, a pathway to violence.* Retrieved from http://www.cchla.ufpb.br/rbse/HartleyArt.pdf

Isiugo-Abanihe, U. C. (2003). *Male role and responsibility in fertility and reproductive health in Nigeria.* Retrieved from http://www.worldcat.org/title/male-role-and-responsibility-in--fertility-and-reproductive-health-in-nigeria/oclc/54042707

Joint United Nations Programme on HIV/AIDS (UNAIDS). (2014a). *The gap report.* Geneva: UNAIDS.

Joint United Nations Programme on HIV/AIDS (UNAIDS). (2014b). *Ending AIDS post-2015: A force for transformation that leaves no one behind.* Retrieved from http://www.unaids.org.cn/en/index/Document_view.asp?id=856

Kyobutungi, C., Ziraba, A. K., Ezeh, A., & Yé, Y. (2008). *The burden of disease profile of residents of Nairobi's slums: Results from a demographic surveillance.* doi:10.1186/1478-7954-6-1.

Luke, N., Xu, H., Mberu, B. U., & Goldberg, R. E. (2012). Migration experience and premarital sexual initiation in urban Kenya: An event history analysis. *Studies in Family Planning, 43*(2), 115–126. Retrieved from http://www.ncbi.nlm.nih.gov/pmc/articles/PMC3665273/

Mberu, B. U. (2012, November 11). *Adolescent sexual and reproductive health and rights: Research evidence from sub-Saharan Africa.* PPD conference "Evidence for action: South-south collaboration for ICPD beyond 2014," Ruposhi Bangla Hotel, Dhaka. Abstract retrieved from http://r4d.dfid.gov.uk/PDF/Outputs/StepUp/2012_PPDMberu.pdf

Mberu, B. U., Mumah, J., Kabiru, C., & Brinton, J. (2014). Bringing sexual and reproductive health in the urban contexts to the forefront of the development Agenda: The case for prioritizing the urban poor. Maternal Child Health, 18(7), 1572–7. doi: 10.1007/s10995-013-1414-7.

National Research Council and Institute of Medicine. (2005). Growing up global: The changing transitions to adulthood in developing countries. In C. B. Lloyd (Ed.), *Growing up global: The changing transitions to adulthood in developing countries.* Washington, DC: The National Academies Press.

Ngware, M., Abuya, B., Admassu, K., Mutisya, M., Musyoka, P., & Oketch, M. (2013). *Quality and access to education in urban informal settlements in Kenya.* Retrieved from http://aphrc.org/publications/quality-and-access-to-education-in-urban-informal-settlements-in-kenya/

Platt, L., Grenfell, P., Fletcher, A., Sorhaindo, A., Jolley, E., Rhodes, T., & Bonell, C. (2013). Systematic review examining differences in HIV, sexually transmitted infection and health-related harms between migrant and non-migrant female sex workers. *Sexually Transmitted Infection, 89*(4), 311–319. doi:10.1136/sextrans-2012-050491.

Richter, M., Chersich, M. F., Vearey, J., Sartorious, B., Temmerman, M., & Luchters, S. (2014). Migration status, work conditions and health utilization of female sex workers in three South African cities. *Journal of Immigration Minor Health, 16*(1), 7–17. doi:10.1007/s10903-012-9758-4.

Ross, C. E., & Mirowsky, J. (2011). Neighborhood disadvantage, disorder and health. *Journal of Health and Social Behavior, 42*(3), 258–276. Retrieved from http://www.jstor.org/stable/3090214

Samson, A. (Ed.). (2014). *The behavioral economics guide 2014* (1st ed.). Retrieved from http://www.behavioraleconomics.com

Slap, G. B., Lucy, L., Damiyam, C. A., Zink, T. M., & Succop, P. A. (2003). Sexual behavior of adolescents in Nigeria: Cross sectional survey of secondary school students. *International Family Planning Perspectives, 23*(1): 28–33. doi:http://dx.doi.org/10.1136/bmj.326.7379.15.

Smith, D. P., & King, R. (2011). Editorial introduction: Re-making migration theory. (Special issue: Re-making migration theory: Transitions, intersections and cross-fertilisations). *Populations, Space and Place, 18*(2), 127–133. doi:10.1002/psp.686.

Spiegel, P. B., Schilperoord, M., & Dahab, M. (2014). High-risk sex and displacement among refugees and surrounding populations in 10 countries: The need for integrating interventions. *AIDS, 28*(5), 761–771. doi:10.1097/QAD.0000000000000118.

United Nations Human Settlements Programme (UN–Habitat). (2006). *Nairobi: Urban sector profile*. Retrieved from http://unhabitat.org/

References

Abma, J., & Sonenstein, F. L. (2001). Sexual activity and contraceptive practices among teenagers in the United States, 1988 and 1995. *Vital and Health Statistics, 23*(21), 1–79. Retrieved from www.cdc.gov/nchs/products/series/series23.htm

Abu, S., Quader, A., Gouws-Williams, E., Tlou, S., Wright-De Agüero, L., & Needle, R. (2015). Key population in sub-Saharan Africa: HIV prevalence, HIV risk behaviours and population size. *AIDS and Behaviour, 19*(1 Suppl 1090–7165), 46–58.

Abuya, B. (2013). *Ministry of Education to reduce the incidence of sexual harassment and violence among girls attending high schools in Kenya by 2015*. Retrieved from www.aphrc.org

Adedimeji, A. A. (2005). *Beyond knowledge and behaviour change: The social-structural context of HIV/AIDS risk perceptions and protective behavior among young urban slum inhabitants in Nigeria*. Retrieved from http://www.einstein.yu.edu/faculty/12079/adebola-adedimeji/

Adetunji, J., & Meekers, D. (2001). Consistency of condom use in the context of AIDS in Zimbabwe. *Journal of Biosocial Science, 33*(1), 121–138. Retrieved from http://www.ncbi.nlm.nih.gov/pubmed/11316390

African Population and Health Research Center. (2013, December 7). *A conceptual framework for UNAIDS/UN-Habitat joint publication on HIV in cities final report*. Unpublished raw data.

African Union. (2011). *The AU's Africa's common position to the high level meeting of the UN General Assembly special session on AIDS*. Retrieved from https://www.google.com/url?sa=t&rct=j&q=&esrc=s

Agostini, G., Chianese, F., French, W., & Sandhu, A. (2006). *Understanding the processes of urban violence*. Retrieved from https://www.eisf.eu/wp-content/uploads/2014/09/0107-Agostini-et-al-2010-Understanding-the-process-of-urban-violence-an-analytical-framework.pdf

Ahlawat, K. A., & Mohammad, S. (1988). Gender and the subjective meaning of health: An integrated approach. *Quality & Quantity: International Journal of Methodology, 22*(2), 151–165.

Ainsworth, M., & Filmer, D. (2002). *Poverty, AIDS and children's schooling: A targeting dilemma* (World Bank Policy Research Working Paper No. 2885). Retrieved from http://documents.worldbank.org/curated/en/2002/09/2017579/poverty-aids-childrens-schooling-targeting-dilemma

All About Nairobi. (2015). *Nairobi slums*. Retrieved from http://www.all-about-nairobi.com/nairobi-slums.html

Amee, S. M. S., Schwitters, A., Swaminathan, M., Serwadda, D., Muyonga, D., Shiraishi, R. W., Benech, I., Mital, S., Bosa, R., Lubwama, G., & Hladik, W. (2015). Prevalence of rape and client-initiated gender-based violence among female sex workers: Kampala, Uganda, 2012. *AIDS and Behaviour, 19*(1), 68–76. doi:10.1007/s10461-014-0957-y.

Andrews, G. S. (2006). Epidemiology of health and vulnerability among children orphaned and made vulnerable by HIV/AIDS in sub-Saharan Africa. *AIDS Care, 18*(3), 269–276.

Anti-Virus Emergency Response Team. (2014a). *HIV/AIDS in Kenya*. Retrieved from http://www.avert.org/hiv-aids-kenya.html

Anti-Virus Emergency Response Team. (2014b). *HIV/AIDS in sub Saharan Africa*. Retrieved from http://www.avert.org/hiv-aids-sub-saharan-africa.htm

Anti-Virus Emergency Response Team. (2014c). *Women and HIV/AIDS*. Retrieved from http://www.avert.org/women-and-hiv-aids.htm

Araya, T., Tensou, B., Davey, G., & Berhane, Y. (2012). Accuracy of physicians in diagnosing HIV/AIDS-related death in the adult population of Addis Ababa, Ethiopia. *World Journal of AIDS, 2*(2), 89–96. doi:10.4236/wja.2012.22012.

Arnold, C., Theede, J., & Gagnon, A. (2014). A qualitative exploration of access to urban migrant healthcare in Nairobi, Kenya. *Social Science and Medical Journal, 110*, 1–9.

Auvert, B., Buvé, A., Ferry, B., Caraël, M., Ary, D., Duncan, T. E., Duncan, S. C., & Hops, H. (1999). Adolescent problem behavior: The influence of parents and peers. *Behaviour Research and Therapy, 37*(3), 217–230. doi:10.1016/S0005-7967(98)00133-8.

Baggaley, R. F., Ferguson, N. M., & Garnett, G. P. (2005). The epidemiological impact of antiretroviral use predicted by mathematical models: A review. *Emerging Themes in Epidemiology, 2*, 9. doi:10.1186/1742-7622-2-9.

Ballard, T., Coates, J., Swindale, A., & Deitchler, M. (2011). *Household hunger scale: Indicator definition and measurement guide*. Washington, DC: Food and Nutrition Technical Assistance II Project (FANTA-2) Bridge, FHI 360.

Bandura, A. (1977). Towards a unifying theory of behavioural change. *Psychology Review, 84*(2), 191–215.

Bankole, A., Darroch, J. E., & Singh, S. (1999). Determinants of trend in condom use in the United States, 1988–1995. *Family Planning Perspectives, 31*(6), 264–271.

Bankole, A., Oye-Adeniran, B. A., Singh, S., Adewole, I. F., Wulf, D., Sedgh, G., & Hussain, R. (2006). Unwanted pregnancy and induced abortion in Nigeria: Causes and consequences. *Journal of Reproductive Health Matters, 15*(29), 231. Retrieved from http://www.guttmacher.org/pubs/2006/08/08/Nigeria-UP-IA.pdf

Bastos, F. I., de Barradas Barata, R., Aquino, E. M., & do Latorre, M. (2008). *Sexual behavior of Brazilian Population and perceptions on HIV/AIDS*. Brasillia: Rev. Saúde Pública.

Bauck, H. (2007). *City guide to Nairobi-The green city in the sun*. Retrieved from Bauck.com: http://www.bauck.com/nairobi-city-guide-green-city-sun/

Berger, P. L., & Luckmann, T. (1966). *The social construction of reality*. New York: Doubleday.

Berquo, E., & Cavengh, S. (1999). *Adolescents, youth and the national demographic health survey*. Retrieved from http://www.stat.go.jp/english/info/148.htm

Birdthistle, I., Floyd, S., Nyagadza, A., Mudziwapasi, N., Gregson, S., & Glynn, J. R. (2009). Is education the link between orphanhood and HIV/HSV-2 risk among female adolescents in urban Zimbabwe? *Social Science and Medicine, 68*(10), 1810–1818.

Black, S. R., & Bull, S. (2013). Actual versus perceived peer sexual risk behavior in online youth social networks. *Translational Behavioral Medicine: Practice, Policy, Research, 3*, 227. doi:10.1007/s13142-013-0227-y.

Blake, J. (1981). Family size and the quality of children. *Demography, 18*(4), 421–442.

Blanc, A. K. (1998). Sexual behavior and contraceptive knowledge and use among adolescents in developing countries. *Studies in Family Planning, 29*(2), 106–116.

Blum, R. W., McNeely, C., & Nonnemaker, J. (2002). Vulnerability, risk and perception. *Journal of Adolescent Health, 31*(1), 28–39. Retrieved from http://www.popline.org/node/242403

Blumenthal, S. (2014). *A world without AIDS for American women*. America Foundation for AIDS Research. Retrieved from http://www.amfar.org/world-without-aids-for-american-women/

Bongaarts, J., Pelletier, F., & Garland, P. (2009). *Poverty, gender and youth. Global trends in AIDS mortality* (Working Paper No. 16). New York: Population Council.

Brewster, K. L., Cooksey, E. C., Guilkey, D. K., & Rinfuss, R. R. (1998). The changing impact of religion on the sexual and contraceptive behavior of adolescent women in the U.S. *Journal of Marriage and the Family, 60*(2), 493–504.

Brokerhoff, M., & Yang, X. (1994). Impact of migration on fertility in sub-Saharan Africa. *Social Biology, 41*(1–2), 19–43.

Brookings Institute. (2010). *IASC framework on durable solutions for internally displaced persons*. University of Bern Project on Internal Displacement. Retrieved from www.brookings.edu/research/reports/2010/03/05-internal-displacement

Busza, J. R., Balakireva, O. M., Teltschik, A., Bondar, T. V., Sereda, Y. V., Meynell, C., & Sakovych, O. (2010). Street- based adolescents at high risk of HIV in Ukraine. *Journal of Epidemiology Community Health, 65*(12), 1166–1170. doi:10.1136/jech.2009.097469.

Butler, C. (2000). HIV/AIDS, poverty and causation. *The Lancet, 356*(9239), 1445–1446. doi:http://dx.doi.org/10.1016/S0140-6736(05)74091-5

Byass, P. (2007). Who needs cause-of-death data? *PLoS Medicine, 4*(11), 333. doi:10.1371/journal.pmed.0040333.

Byass, P., Berhane, Y., Emmelin, A., Kebede, D., Andersson, T., Högberg, U., & Wall, S. (2002). The role of demographic surveillance systems (DSS) in assessing the health of communities: An example from rural Ethiopia. *Public Health, 116*(3), 145–150.

Caldwell, J. (2000). Rethinking the African AIDS epidemic. *Population Development Review, 26*(1), 117–135. doi:10.1111/j.1728-4457.2000.00117.x.

Caritas. (2008, September 13–15). *Caritas Africa forum, Addis Ababa, Ethiopia*. Retrieved from http://www.caritas-africa.org/2008forumeng.pdf.

Center for Security Studies. (2013). *The CSS analysis* (Security Policy 142). Zurich: Centre for Security Studies.

Chambers, R. (1983). *Rural development: Putting the last first*. Harlow: Longman.

Chege, F. N., & Sifuna, D. N. (2006). *Girls and women's education in Kenya: Gender perspectives and trends*. Retrieved from http://ir-library.ku.ac.ke/handle/123456789/8484

Chege, M. N., Kabiru, E. W., Mbithi, J. N., & Bwayo, J. J. (2002). Childcare practices of commercial sex workers. *East Africa Medical Journal, 79*(7), 382–389.

Cheru, F. (2002). *African renaissance: Roadmaps to the challenge of globalization*. London and New York: Zed Books. Zed Books. doi: 10.2307/3556919; 10.107/S0022278X04214446.

Chirwa, W. C. (1997). Migrant labour, sexual networking and multi-partnered sex in Malawi. *Health Transition Review, 7*(Suppl 3), 5–15. Retrieved from http://htc.anu.edu.au/pdfs/Chirwa1.pdf

Chukwuezi, B. (2001). Through thick and thin: Igbo rural–urban circularity, identity and investment. *Journal of Contemporary African Studies, 19*(1), 55–66.

Clayton, R. R. (1980). Premarital sex in the seventies. *Journal of Marriage and Family, 42*(4), 759–775. doi:10.2307/351823.

Cloutier, S., Martin, S. L., & Pool, C. (2002). Sexual assault among North Carolina women: Prevalence and health risk factors. *Journal of Epidemiology & Community Health, 56*, 265–271. doi:10.1136/jech.56.4.265.

Cluver, L., & Operario, D. (2009). Inter-generational linkages of AIDS: Vulnerability of orphaned children for HIV infection. *IDS Bulletin, 39*(5), 27. doi:10.1111/j.1759-5436.2008.tb00492.x.

Coalition of Violence Against Women Kenya. (2008). *Rapid assessment of the situation of displaced women and girls in Western Kenya: Kisumu, Kakamega and Kisii*. Retrieved from COVAWK website: www.peacewomen.org/portal resources resources.php?id=24

Cohen, A. (2003). *Urban unfinished business*. doi:10.2307/3342681.

Cohen, J. H. (2004). *The culture of migration in Southern Mexica*. Retrieved from http://utpress.utexas.edu/index.php/books/cohcul

Cooksey, E. R. (1996). The initiation of adolescent sexual and contraceptive behavior during changing times. *Journal of Health and Social Behaviors, 37*, 59–74. Retrieved from http://www.jstor.org/stable/2137231

Copas, A. J., McManus, S., Wellings, K., Fenton, K. A., Korovessis, C., Macdowall, W., Nanchahal, K., Purdon, S., & Field, J. (2001). Sexual behaviour in Britain: Partnerships, practices, and HIV risk behaviours. *The Lancet, 358*(9296), 1835–1842. doi:10.1016/S0140-6736(01)06883-0.

Craddock, S. (2001). Women, inequity, and AIDS in East Africa. In I. Dyck, N. Lewis, & A. N. MacLafferty (Eds.), *Geographies of women's health*. London/New York: Routledge.

Creswell, J. W., & Plano Clark, V. L. (2011). *Designing and conducting mixed methods research.* Los Angeles: SAGE Publications.

Da Silva, D., Joseph, D., Gune, E., Mussá, F., Wheeler, J., Benedetti, M., & Chissano, M. (2010). *Study about vulnerability and risk to HIV infection among men who have sex with men in Maputo city.* USAID.

Dahab, M., Spiegel, P. B., Njogu, P. M., & Schilperoord, M. (2013). Changes in HIV-related behaviours, knowledge and testing among refugees and surrounding national populations: A multicountry study. *AIDS Care, 25*(8), 998–1009. doi:10.1080/09540121.2012.748165.

Danziger, S. H., & Haveman, R. H. (Eds.). (2001). *Understanding poverty.* New York: Russell Sage Foundation.

Davidson, J. K. (1977). Premarital sexual intercourse: An application of axiomatic theory constriction. *Journal of Marriage and Family, 39,* 15–25. Retrieved from http://eric.ed.gov/?id=EJ154686

Davinder, L. (1994). The forgotten half: Environment health in Nairobi's poverty areas. *Environment and Urbanization, 6,* 164–168.

De la Barra, X. (1998). Poverty: The main cause of ill health in urban children. *Health Education and Behaviour, 25*(1), 46–59. Retrieved from http://www.popline.org/node/273984

Dunne, M., Humphreys, S., & Leach, F. (2003). *Gender and violence in schools. Background paper prepared for the education for all global monitoring report 2003/4: Gender and education for all: The leap to equality.* Retrieved from: http://www.popline.org/node/276312#sthash.Ltf2Zxvs.dpuf

Emmanuel, M., & Yarime, M. (2011). Understanding the grassroots dynamics of slums in Nairobi: The dilemma of Kibera informal settlements. *International Transaction Journal of Engineering, Management, & Applied Sciences & Technologies.* Retrieved from http://tuengr.com/V02/197-213.pdf

Environmental Change and Security Programme. (2005). *Growing up global: The changing transition to adulthood in developing countries.* Washington, DC: National Academic Press.

Epstein, H. (2014). *The missing science. Uganda's anti gay law.* Retrieved from http://www.nybooks.com/blogs/nyrblog/2014/feb/26/uganda-anti-gay-science/

Erikson E. (1950). Childhood and society. In W. E. Roweton (Ed.), *Psychology in the schools, 32*(3), 243. doi:10.1002/1520-6807(199507).

European Coalition of Positive People (ECPP). (1994). *Declaration of the Paris AIDS summit of heads of government on HIV/AIDS.* Retrieved from http://data.unaids.org/pub/ExternalDocument/2007/theparisdeclaration_en.pdf

Ezeh, A. C., Bongaarts, J., & Mberu, B. U. (2012). Global population trends and policy options. *The Lancet, 380*(9837), 142–148. doi:http://dx.doi.org/10.1016/S0140-6736(12)60696-5.

Ferencic, N. E. (2010). *Blame and Banishment: The underground HIV epidemic affecting children in Eastern Europe and Central Asia.* Geneva: UNICEF.

Fotso, J. C. (2008). Urban–rural differentials in child malnutrition in sub-Saharan Africa: Trends and socioeconomic correlates. *Health Places, 13,* 205–223. Retrieved from http://www.ncbi.nlm.nih.gov/pubmed/16563851

Fotso, J. C., Cleland, J., Mberu, B., Mutua, M., & Elungata, P. (2012). Birth spacing and child mortality: An analysis of prospective data from the Nairobi Urban Health and Demographic Surveillance System. *Journal of Biosocial Science, 45*(6), 779–798. doi:10.1017/S0021932012000570.

French, D. C., & Dishion, T. (2003). Predictors of early initiation of sexual intercourse among high-risk adolescents. *The Journal of Early Adolescence, 23*(3):295–315. Retrieved from Sage Journals: http://jea.sagepub.com/content/23/3/295.abstract

Gadin, K. G., & Hammarström, A. (2003). Do changes in the psychosocial school environment influence pupils health development? Result from a three year follow up study Scandinavian. *Journal of Public Health, 31,* 169–177. Retrieved from http://sjp.sagepub.com/content/31/3/169.abstract

Galloway, M. (2015, May). City slums: a big health risk in southern Africa. *SciBraai.* Retrieved from http://aphrc.org/city-slums-a-big-health-risk-in-southern-africa/

Galtung, J. (1969). Violence, peace, and peace research. *Journal of Peace Research, 6*(3), 167–191. Retrieved from http://www.jstor.org/stable/422690

Garcia-Moreno, C., Heise, L., Jansen, H. A., Ellsberg, M., & Watts, C. (2005). Public health: Violence against women. *Science, 310*(5752), 1282–1283. Retrieved from http://www.ncbi. nlm.nih.gov/pubmed/16311321

Garmezy, N. (1991). Resilience and vulnerability to adverse developmental outcomes associated with poverty. *American Behavioural Sciences, 4*(34), 416–430. doi:10.1177/0002764291034004003.

Gelmon, L., Kenya, P., Oguya, F., Chelugat, B., & Haile, G. (2009a). *HIV prevention response and modes of transmission analysis* (Final Report). Retrieved from http://siteresources.worldbank. org/INTHIVAIDS/Resources/375798-1103037153392/KenyaMOT22March09Final.pdf

George, M. (2007). *State of the world population: Unleashing the potential of urban growth.* New York: UNFPA.

Geschiere, P., & Gugler, J. (1998). The urban–rural connections: Changing issues of belonging and identification. *Africa, 68*(3), 309–319. doi:http://dx.doi.org/10.2307/1161251.

Ghosh, J., Wadhwa, V., & Kalipeni, E. (2009). Vulnerability to HIV/AIDS among women of reproductive age in the slums of Delhi and Hyderabad. *Social Science and Medicine, 68*(4), 638–642. doi:10.1016/j.socscimed.2008.11.023.

Goffman, E. (1959). *Presentation of self in everyday life.* New York: Doubleday.

Goldberg, R. F. (2013). Family instability and early initiation of sexual activity in western Kenya. *Demography, 50*(2), 725–750. doi:10.1007/s13524-012-0150-8.

Government of Kenya. (2007). *National plan for orphans and vulnerable children.* Nairobi: Government of Kenya.

Government of Kenya. (2012). *Education medium term expenditure framework* (Sector Report: 2013/14- 2015/16). Nairobi: Government of Kenya.

Grotberg, E. H. (1994). A guide to promoting resilience in children: Strengthening the human spirit. In *Early childhood development: Practice and reflections* series (Vol. 8). Retrieved from http://www.scribd.com/doc/143356868/A-Guide-to-Promoting-Resilience-in-Children-Strengthening-the-Human-Spirit#scribdBirmingham

Gugler, J. (1991). Life is a dual system revisited: Urban–rural ties in Enugu, Nigeria 1961–87. *World Development, 19*(5), 399–409. Retrieved from http://www.sciencedirect.com/science/article/pii/0305750X9190185K

Guo, G., & Harris, K. M. (1999). The mechanics mediating the effects of poverty on children's intellectual development. *Demography, 37*(4), 431–447. Retrieved from http://www.ncbi.nlm. nih.gov/pubmed/11086569

Guru, G. (Ed.). (2009). *Humiliation: Claims and context.* Oxford: Oxford University Press.

Harris, B., Goudge, J., Ataguba, J. E., McIntyre, D., Nxumalo, N., Jikwana, S., & Chersich, M. (2011). Inequalities in access to health care in South Africa. *Journal of Public Health Policy, 32*, 102–123. doi:10.1057/jphp.2011.35.

Hartling, L., & Luchetta, T. (1999). Humiliation: Assessing the impact of derision, degradation, and debasement. *Journal of Primary Prevention, 19*(4), 259–278. doi:10.1023/A:1022622422521.

Hater, S. (1987). The perceived competence scale for children. *Child Development, 53*(1), 8797. doi:10.2307/1129640.

Hayase, Y., & Liaw, K. L. (1997). Factors on polygamy in sub-Saharan Africa: Findings based on the demographic and health surveys. *The Developing Economies, 35*(3), 293–327. Retrieved from http://www.ncbi.nlm.nih.gov/pubmed/12293108

Herbst, A. J., Cooke, G. S., Bärnighausen, T., KanyKany, A., Tanser, F., & Newell, M. L. (2009). Adult mortality and antiretroviral treatment roll-out in rural Kwazulu-Natal, South Africa. *Bulletin of the World Health Organisation, 87*(10), 754–762. Retrieved from http://www.ncbi. nlm.nih.gov/pubmed/19876542

Hervitz, H. M. (1985). Selectivity, adaptation or disruption? A comparison of alternative hypotheses on the effects of migration on fertility: The case of Brazil. *International Migration Review, 19*(2), 293–317. Retrieved from http://www.popline.org/node/417542

Hindin, M. J., & Fatusi, A. O. (2009). Adolescent sexual and reproductive health and rights: Research evidence from sub-Saharan Africa. *International Perspective on Sexual and Reproductive Health, 35*(2). doi: 10.1363/3505809.

Howard, B. H., Phillips, C. V., Matinhure, N., Goodman, K. J., McCurdy, S. A., & Johnson, C. A. (2006). Barriers and incentives to orphan care in a time of AIDS and economic crisis: A cross-sectional survey of caregivers in the rural Zimbabwe. *Biological Medicine Central, Public Health, 6*(1), 27. doi:10.1186/1471-2458-6-27.

Igwe, A. N. (2004). *Abortion among non-school youths in Nigeria.* Retrieved from http://paa2004. princeton.edu/papers/40125

Inter Agency Standing Committee on HIV in Emergencies. (2010). *Guidelines for addressing HIV in humanitarian settings.* Geneva: UNAIDS.

Internal Displacement Monitoring Centre. (2008). *A profile of the internal displaced situation.* Retrieved from http://www.internal-displacemnt.org/

International Labour Office. (2012). *The youth unemployment crisis: Time for action.* Geneva: International Labour Office.

International Organization on Migration and African Population and Health Research Center (2015). Regional synthesis on patterns and determinants of migrants' health and associated vulnerabilities in urban setting of East and Southern Africa. Johannesburg: International Organization on Migration.

Iqbal, Z., & Zorn, C. (2010). Violent conflict and the spread of HIV/AIDS in Africa. *The Journal of Politics, 72*(1), 149–162. doi:http://dx.doi.org/10.1017/S0022381609990533.

Irwin, A., Adams, A., & Winter, A. (2009). Home truths: Facing the facts on children, AIDS, and poverty. In A. Irwin, A. Adams, & A. Winter (Eds.), *Joint learning initiative on children* (p. 84). Retrieved from http://www.jlica.org/protected/pdf-feb09/Final%20J

Isiugo-Abanihe, I. M. (2005). *Benefits of sexuality education for young persons in Nigeria.* Retrieved from http://www.arsrc.org/downloads/uhsss/ajuwon.pdf

Isiugo-Abanihe, U. C., & Oyediran, K. (2004). Household socioeconomic status and sexual behaviour among Nigerian female youth. *African Population Studies, 19*(1), 81–98.

Itaborahy, L. P., & Zhu, J. (2013). *State-sponsored homophobia – A world survey of laws: Criminalization, protection and recognition of same-sex love.* Retrieved from The International Lesbian, Gay, Bisexual, Trans and Intersex Association website: www.ilga.org

Jahn, A., Floyd, S., Crampin, A. C., Mwaungulu, F., Mvula, H., Munthali, F., McGrath, N., Mwafilaso, J., Mwinuka, V., Mangongo, B., Fine, P. E. M., Zaba, B., & Glynn, R. J. (2008). Population-level effect of HIV on adult mortality and early evidence of reversal after introduction of antiretroviral therapy in Malawi. *Lancet, 371*(9624), 1603–1611. doi:10.1016/S0140-6736(08)60693-5.

Jamison, D. T., Breman, J. G., Measham, A. R., Alleyne, G., Claeson, M., Evans, D. B., Jha, P., Mills, A., & Musgrove, P. (Eds.). (2006). *Disease control priorities in developing countries* (2nd ed.). Washington, DC: Oxford University Press.

Jessor, R. (1992). Risk behaviour in adolescence: A psychosocial framework for understanding and action. *Developmental Review, 12*(4), 374–390. Retrieved from http://www.sciencedirect. com/science/article/pii/027322979290014S

Jessor, R., Turbin, M. S., & Costa, F. M. (1998). Protective factors in adolescents health behaviour. *Journal of Personality and Social Psychology, 75*(30), 788–800. doi:http://dx.doi. org/10.1037/0022-3514.75.3.788.

Jewkes, R. K., Dunkle, K., Nduna, M., & Shai, M. (2010). Intimate partner violence, relationship power inequity, and incidence of HIV infection in young women in South Africa: A cohort study. *The Lancet, 376*(9734), 41–48. doi:10.1016/S0140-6736(10)60548-X.

Joint United Nations Programme on HIV/AIDS (UNAIDS). (1996). *Global strategy.* Retrieved from http://data.unaids.org/publications/irc-pub01/jc208-corpreport_en.pdf

Joint United Nations Programme on HIV/AIDS (UNAIDS). (2008, May). *Facts about HIV.* Retrieved from http://data.unaids.org/pub/FactSheet/2008/20080519_fastfacts_hiv_en.pdf

Joint United Nations Programme on HIV/AIDS (UNAIDS). (2012a). *Global AIDS report 2012.* Geneva: UNAIDS.

Joint United Nations Programme on HIV/AIDS (UNAIDS). (2012b). *The UNAIDS agenda for accelerated country action for women, girls, gender, equality and AIDS (AACA)* (Mid-Term Review – Final Report). Retrieved from http://www.unaids.org/sites/default/files/sub_landing/ files/20121206_Final_Report_Mid_Term%20Review_UNAIDS_Agenda_for_Women_and_ Girls.pdf

Joint United Nations Programme on HIV/AIDS (UNAIDS). (2014f, July 16). *UNAIDS report shows 19 million of the 35 million people living with HIV today do not know that they have the virus.* Retrieved from http://www.unaids.org/en/resources/presscentre/pressreleaseandstatementarchive/2014/july/20140716prgareport

Joint United Nations Programme on HIV/AIDS (UNAIDS). (2014g). *Progress report on the global plan. Towards the elimination of new HIV infections among children by 2015 and keeping their mothers alive* (Report No. JC2681/1/E). Geneva: UNAIDS.

Joint United Nations Programme on HIV/AIDS (UNAIDS) & World Health Organization (WHO). (2006). *AIDS epidemic update.* Geneva: WHO.

Jones, R. K., Darroch, J. E., & Singh, S. (2005). Religious differentials in the sexual and reproductive behaviors of young women in the United States. *Journal of Adolescents Health, 36*(4), 279–288. doi:10.1016/j.jadohealth.2004.02.036.

Kabiru, C. W., Beguy, B., Crichton, J., & Zulu, E. M. (2011). HIV/AIDS among youth in urban informal (slum) settlements in Kenya: What are the correlates of and motivations for HIV testing? *BioMed Centre, Public Health, 11*, 685. doi:10.1186/1471-2458-11-685.

Kahn, K., Tollman, S. M., Garenne, M., & Gear, J. S. (2000). Validation and application of verbal autopsies in rural areas of South Africa. *Tropical Medical and International Health, 5*(11), 824–831.

Kamau, N., & Esamai, F. O. (2001). Determinants of immunisation coverage among children in Mathare Valley, Nairobi. *East African Medical Journal, 78*(11), 590–594. Retrieved from http://www.ncbi.nlm.nih.gov/pubmed/12219965

Kambarami, M. (2006). *Feminity, sexuality and culture: Patriarchy and females subordination in Zimbabwe.* Retrieved from http://www.arsrc.org/downloads/uhsss/kmabarami.pdf

Karimi, F., & Dutheris, V. (2014, January 16). Nigeria arrests gay suspects under new law banning homosexuality. *Cable Network News.* Retrieved from http://edition.cnn.com/2014/01/16/world/africa/nigeria-anti-gay-law-arrests/index.html

Kariuki, C. (2004). *Masculinity and adolescents male violence: The case of three secondary schools in Kenya.* Retrieved from http://aphrc.org/

Kenya National AIDS Control Council (NACC) & Office of the President. (2008). *UNGASS 2008 country report for Kenya.* Nairobi: Kenya National AIDS Control Council.

Kenya National AIDS Control Council (NACC), & Kenya National AIDS & STI Control Programme (NASCOP). (2012). *The Kenya AIDS epidemic update, 2012.* Nairobi: National AIDS Control Council & Kenya National AIDS & STI Control Programme.

Kenya National AIDS Control Council (NACC), & Ministry of Health Kenya & Joint United Nations Programme on HIV/AIDS (UNAIDS). (2014). *HIV and AIDS profile Nairobi County, Kenya, 2014.* Nairobi: Kenya National AIDS Control Council.

Kenya National AIDS Control Council (NACC), Joint United Nations Programme on HIV/AIDS (UNAIDS), & The World Bank Global HIV/AIDS Program. (2009). *Kenya HIV prevention response and modes of transmission analysis final report.* Retrieved from http://siteresources.worldbank.org/INTHIVAIDS/Resources/375798-1103037153392/KenyaMOT22March09Final.pdf

Kenya National Bureau of Statistics. (2009). *Population and housing census.* Retrieved from http://www.knbs.or.ke/index.php?option=com_phocadownload&view=category&id=109:population-and-housing-census-2009&itemid=599

Kenya National Data Archive (KeNADA). (2015). *Kenya – Kenya AIDS indicator survey.* Retrieved from http://statistics.knbs.or.ke/nada/index.php

Kenya National AIDS and STI Control Programme (NASCOP). (2011). *Kenya HIV drug resistance country report 2010–2011.* Retrieved from www.nascop.or.ke

Kenya National AIDS & STI Control Programme (NASCOP). (2012). *HIV testing and counselling.* Retrieved from http://nascop.org/nascop/hiv_testing_&_counselling.html

Kenya National AIDS and STI Control Programme (NASCOP), Centre for Disease Control (CDC) Kenya, Centers for Disease Control and Prevention (U.S.), Joint United Nations Programme on HIV/AIDS (UNAIDS); United States, Agency for International Development (UNAIDS), & U.S. President's Emergency Plan for AIDS Relief & World Health Organization. (2009). *2007 Kenya AIDS indicator survey; KAIS 2007: Final report.* Retrieved from www.nascop.or.ke

Kenya National AIDS and STI Control Programme (NASCOP), Centre for Disease Control (CDC) Kenya, Centers for Disease Control and Prevention (U.S.), Joint United Nations Programme on

HIV/AIDS (UNAIDS); United States, Agency for International Development (UNAIDS), & U.S. President's Emergency Plan for AIDS Relief. (2014a). *Kenya AIDS indicator survey 2012: Final report.* Retrieved from www.nascop.or.ke

Kenya National AIDS & STI Control Programme (NASCOP) & Ministry of Health. (2013, September). *Kenya AIDS Indicator Survey 2012: Preliminary Report.* Nairobi: National AIDS & STI Control Programme.

Kenya National AIDS & STI Control Programme (NASCOP), & Ministry of Health. (2013a). *Kenya most at risk population size estimate consensus report.*

Kenya National AIDS & STI Control Programme (NASCOP), & Ministry of Health. (2013b, September). *Kenya AIDS indicator survey 2012: Preliminary report.* Retrieved from http://www.scribd.com/doc/167580994/Preliminary-Report-for-Kenya-AIDS-indicator-survey-2012-pdf#scribd

Kenya National AIDS & STI control Programme (NASCOP), Kenya National AIDS Control Council (NACC) & Joint United Nations Programme on HIV/AIDS (UNAIDS). (2015). *HIV/AIDS in Kenya 2014 Fact sheet.* Nairobi: National AIDS Control Council of Kenya

Kenya National AIDS & STI Control Programme (NASCOP), Kenya National AIDS Control Council (NACC), & Liverpool Voluntary Counselling and Testing (LVCT) & United Nations Children's Fund (UNICEF). (2015). *Adolescents, youth and HIV in Kenya, 2014, fact sheet.* Nairobi: Kenya National AIDS Control Programme

Kenya National AIDS & STI Control Programme (NASCOP), Kenya National AIDS Control Council (NACC), & Liverpool Voluntary Counselling and Testing (LVCT) & United Nations Children's Fund (UNICEF). (2014b). *Adolescents, youth and HIV in Kenya, 2014, fact sheet.*

Kimani-Murage, E. W., Holding, P. A., Fotso, J. C., Ezeh, A. C., & Madise, N. J. (2008). Food security and nutritional outcomes of urban poor orphaned children in Nairobi. *Journal of Urban Health: Bulletin of the New York Academy of Medicine, 88*(2), 282–295. doi:10.1007/s11524-010-9491-z.

Knodel, J., & Van de Walle, E. (1979). Lessons from the past: Policy implications of historical fertility studies. *Population and Development Review, 5*(2), 217–245.

Kouyoumdjian, F. G., Calzavara, L. M., Bondy, S. J., O'Campo, P., Serwadda, D., Nalugoda, F., Kagaayi, J., Kigozi, G., Wawer, M., & Gray, R. (2013). Intimate partner violence is associated with incidence HIV infection in women in Uganda. *AIDS, 27*(8), 1331–1338. doi:10.1097/QAD.0b013e32835fd851.

Kraus, S. J. (2014, July). *Place matters: Why cities are key to ending AIDS cities for social transformation towards ending AIDS. UNAIDS.* Paper presented at the 20th international AIDS conference, Melbourne. Retrieved from http://www.aidsdatahub.org

Krieger, N., Williams, R., & Moss, N. E. (1997). Measuring social class in US Public Health Research: Concepts, methodology, and guidelines. *Annual Review of Public Health, 18*, 341–378.

Ku, L., Sonenstein, F. L., & Pleck, J. H. (1992). Patterns of HIV risk and preventive behaviors among teenage men. *Public Health Reports, 107*(2), 131–138. Retrieved from http://www.jstor.org/stable/4597090

Kubler-Ross, E. (1997). *On death and dying.* London/New York: Routledge.

Lagarde, E. M., Schim van der Loeff, M., Enel, C., Holmgren, B., Dray-Spira, R., Pison, G., Piau, J. P., Delaunay, V., M'Boup, S., Ndoye, I., Cœuret-Pellicer, M., Whittle, H., & Aaby, P. (2003). Mobility and the spread of human immunodeficiency virus into rural areas of West Africa. *International Journal of Epidemiology, 32*(5), 744–752. Retrieved from http://www.ncbi.nlm.nih.gov/pubmed/14559743

Langford, M., & Du Plessis, J. (2009). *Dignity in the rubble? Forced evictions and human rights law.* Retrieved from https://www.jus.uio.no/smr/english/people/aca/malcolml/dignity-in-the-rubble-human-rights-law-and-forced-evictions.pdf

Lazano, R., et al. (2012). Global and regional mortality from 235 causes of death for 20 age groups in 1990 and 2010: A systematic analysis for the global burden of disease study 2010. *The Lancet, 380*(9859), 2095–2128. doi:http://dx.doi.org/10.1016/S0140-6736(12)61728-0.

Lee, B. S., & Farber, S. C. (1984). Fertility adaptation by rural–urban migrants in developing countries: The case of Korea. *Population Studies, 38*(1), 141–156. doi:10.2307/2174360.

Lescano, C. M., Vazquez, E. A., Brown, L. K., Litvin, E. B., Pugatch, D., & Project SHIELD Study Group. (2006). Condom use with casual and main partners: What's in a name? *Journal of Adolescent Health, 39*, 443–447. doi:http://dx.doi.org/10.1016/j.jadohealth.2006.01.003.

Li, X., Stanton, B., & Feigelman, S. (1999). Exposure to drug trafficking among urban, low-income African children and adolescents. *Archives of Pediatric Adolescents Medicine, Journal, 153*(2), 161–168. Retrieved from http://www.ncbi.nlm.nih.gov/pubmed/9988246

Luke, N. (2003). Age and economics asymmetries in the sexual relationship of adolescents girls in sub-Saharan Africa. *Studies in Family Planning, 34*(2), 67–86. doi:10.1111/j.1728-4465.2003.00067.x.

Luke, N. (2010). Migrants' competing commitments: Sexual partners in urban Africa and remittances to the rural origin. *AJS, 115*(5), 1435–1479. Retrieved from http://www.ncbi.nlm.nih.gov/pmc/articles/PMC3728829/

Lurie, M., Harrison, A., Wilkinson, D., & Abdool Karim, S. (1997). Circular migration and sexual networking in Kwazulu Natal: Implications for the spread of HIV and other sexually transmitted diseases. *Health Transition Review, 7*(3), 17–27. Retrieved from http://www.popline.org/node/274510

Lydie, N., Robinson, N. J., Ferry, B., De Loemzien, A. M., Zekeng, L., & Abega, S. (2004). Adolescents sexuality and the HIV epidemic in Yaounde, Cameroon. *Journal of Biosocial Science, 36*(5), 597–616. doi:http://dx.doi.org/DOI:10.1017/S002193200300631X.

Maharaj, P., & Cleland, J. (2005). Risk perception & condom use among married or cohabiting couples in KwaZulu-Natal, South Africa. *International Family Planning Perspectives, 31*(1), 24–29. Retrieved from http://www.ncbi.nlm.nih.gov/pubmed/15888406

Maina, W. K., Kim, A. A., Rutherford, G. W., Harper, M., K'Oyugi, B. O., Sharif, S., Kichamu, G., Muraguri, N. M., Akhwale, W., & De Cock, K. M. (2014). Kenya AIDS indicator surveys 2007 and 2012: Implications for public health policies for HIV prevention and treatment. *Journal of Acquired Immune Deficiency Syndrome, 66*(Suppl 1), 130–137. Retrieved from http://www.medscape.com/medline/abstract/24732817

Manlove, J., Ryan, S., & Franzetta, K. (2003). Patterns of contraceptive use within teenagers first sexual relationship. *Perspectives on Sexual and Reproductive Health, 35*(6), 246–255. doi:10.1363/psrh.35.246.03.

Manlove, J., Moore, K. A., Liechty, J., Ikramullah, E. N., & Cottingham, S. (2005). *Sex between young teens and older individual: A demographic portrait* (Research Brief, No. 2005-07). Retrieved from http://eric.ed.gov/?id=ED486183WashingtonDC

Mann, J. (1998). AIDS and human rights: Where do we go from here? HIV/AIDS and human rights, part ii. *Health and Human Rights, 3*, 143–149. Retrieved from http://www.hhrjournal.org/wp-content/uploads/sites/13/2014/03/9-Mann.pdf

Mann, J., & Tarantola, D. (Eds.). (1992). *AIDS in the World II: Global dimensions, social roots, and responses* (2nd ed., Vol. 2). Cambridge: Harvard University Press.

Manning, W. D., Longmore, M. A., & Giordano, P. C. (2000). The relationship context of contraceptive use at first intercourse. *Family Planning Perspectives, 32*(3), 104–110. Retrieved from http://www.ncbi.nlm.nih.gov/pubmed/10894255

Marshall, S. J. (2004). Developing countries face double burden of disease. *Bulletin of the World Health Organization, 82*(7), 556.

Martin, J. A., Hamilton, B. E., Sutton, P. D., Ventura, S. J., Menacker, F., & Kirmeyer, S. (2006). *Births: Final data for 2004* (National Vital Statistics Report, 55(1)). Retrieved from http://www.cdc.gov/nchs/data/nvsr/nvsr55/nvsr55_01.pdf

Martínez, J., Mboup, G., Sliuzas, R., & Stein, A. (2008). Trends in urban and slum indicators across developing world cities, 1990–2003. *Habitat International, 32*(1), 86–108. doi:10.1016/j.habitatint.2007.08.018.

Mason, K. O. (1995). *Gender demographic change, what do we know?* Retrieved from http://www.popline.org/node/309649

Masten, A. S., Hubbard, J. J., Gest, S. D., Tellegen, A., Garmezy, N., & Ramirez, M. (1999). Competence in the context of adversity: Pathways to resilience and maladaptation from childhood to late adolescence. *Development Psychology, 71*(1), 543–562. Retrieved from http://www.ncbi.nlm.nih.gov/pubmed/10208360

Mathers, C. D., Ma Fat, D., Inoue, M., Rao, C., & Lopez, A. D. (2005). Counting the dead and what they died from: An assessment of the global status of cause of death data. *Bulletin of the World Health Organization, 83*(3), 171–177. Retrieved from http://www.who.int/bulletin/volumes/83/3/mathers0305abstract/en/

Mberu, B. U., & Mutua, M. (2014). Internal migration and early life mortality in Kenya and Nigeria. *Population Place and Space*. doi:10.1002/psp.1857.

Mberu, B. U., Mumah, J., Kabiru, C., & Brinton, J. (2014). Bringing sexual and reproductive health in the urban contexts to the forefront of the development Agenda: The case for prioritizing the urban poor. *Maternal and Child Health, 18*(7), 1572–1577. doi:10.1007/s10995-013-1414-7.

McKenzie, J. (2001). *Changing education: A sociology of education since 1944*. New York: Routledge.

McLeish, K. (1993) *Bloomsbury guide to human thought*. Retrieved from http://books.google.co.ke/books/about/Bloomsbury_Guide_to_Human_Thought.html?id=eDSKQgAACAAJ&redir_esc=y

McMichael, A. (2004). Environmental and social influences on emerging infectious diseases: Past, present and future. *Philosophical Transactions of the Royal Society, London Biological Sciences, 359*(1447), 1049–1058. Retrieved from http://www.ncbi.nlm.nih.gov/pubmed/15306389

McMichael, A. J., & Weiss, R. A. (2004). Social and environment risk factors in the emergence of infectious diseases. *Nature Medicine, 10*(12), 70–6. Retrieved from http://www.ncbi.nlm.nih.gov/pubmed/15577934

McMichael, A. J., McKee, M., Shkolnikov, V., & Valkonen, T. (2004). Mortality trends and set-backs: Global convergence or divergence? *The Lancet, 363*(9415), 1155–1159. doi:10.1016/S0140-6736(04)15902-3.

Michael. (2015). *Life on HIV treatment – A personal perspective by Michael*. Retrieved from NAM AIDSmap: http://www.aidsmap.com/life-on-HIV-treatment-a-personal-perspective/page/1255106/

Milan, S., Zona, K., Acker, J., & Turcios-Cotto, V. (2013). Prospective risk factors for adolescents PTSD: Sources of differential exposure and differential vulnerability. *Journal of Abnormal Child Psychology, 41*(2), 339–353. doi:10.1007/s10802-012-9677.

Miller, B. C., & Moore, K. A. (1990). Adolescent sexual behaviour, pregnancy, and parenting: Research through the 1980's. *Journal of Marriage and Family, 52*(4), 1025–1044. Retrieved from http://www.childtrends.org/?publications=adolescent-sexual-behavior-pregnancy-and-parenting-research-through-the-1980s

Mills, S., Saidel, T., Bennett, A., Rehle, T., Hogle, J., Brown, T., & Magnani, R. (1998). AIDS. HIV risk behavioral surveillance: A methodology for monitoring behavioral trends. *AIDS, 12*(2), 37–46. Retrieved from https://www.researchgate.net/publication/13494770_HIV_risk_behavioral_surveillance_a_methodology_for_monitoring_behavioral_trends

Ministry of Health, Kenya National AIDS Control Council (NACC), Liverpool Voluntary Counselling and Testing (LVCT), Kenya National AIDS & STI Control Programme (NASCOP), & United Nations Children's Fund (UNICEF). (2015). *Adolescents, youth and HIV in Kenya, 2014 fact sheet.*

Minki, C., Murray, N., London, D., & Anglewicz, P. (2004, October). *The factors influencing transactional sex among young men and women in 12 sub-Saharan Africa countries*. Retrieved from http://pdf.usaid.gov/pdf_docs/PNADA925.pdf

Mitullah, W. (2003). *Understanding slums: Case studies for the global report on human settlements. The case of Nairobi, Kenya*. Retrieved from http://www.ucl.ac.uk/dpu-projects/Global_Report/home.htm

Mohamed, A. H., Dalal, W., Nyoka, R., Burke, H., Ahmed, J., Auko, E., Shihaji, W., Ndege, I., Breiman, R. F., & Eidex, R. B. (2014). Health care utilization for acute illnesses in an urban setting with a refugee population in Nairobi, Kenya: A cross- sectional survey. *BioMed Centre, 14*, 200. doi:10.1186/1472-6963-14-200.

Montgomery, M., Stren, R., Cohen, B., & Reed, H. (2003). *Cities transformed: Demographic change and its implications in the developing world*. Washington, DC: National Academic Press.

Morison, L., Lagarde, E., Robinson, N. J., Kahindo, M., Chege, J., Rutenberg, N., Musonda, R., Laourou, M., & Akam, E. (2001). Ecological and individual level analysis of risk factors for HIV infection in four urban populations in sub-Saharan Africa with different levels of HIV infection. *AIDS, 15*(4), 15–30.

Morocco, K. (2013). *Tackling HIV/AIDS among key population, essential to achieving an AIDS – Free generation.* Retrieved from http://amfar.org/uploadedfiles/amfarorg/articles/on the hill/2013/Key%20populations%20issue%20brief%20final%20(2).pdf

Morse, S. (1995). Factors in the emergence of infectious diseases. *Emergence Infectious Diseases, 1,* 7–15. Retrieved from http://wwwnc.cdc.gov/eid/article/1/1/pdfs/95-0102.pdf

Muller, O., & Kwawinkel, M. (2003). Malnutrition and health in developing countries. *Canadian Medical Association Journal, 173*(3), 279–286.

Mzungu, M. (1999, March 6). *Girl domestic workers in Kenya.* Links (Oxford). Retrieved from http://www.ncbi.nlm.nih.gov/pubmed/12295034

Nada, K. H., & El Suliman, D. A. (2010). Violence, abuse, alcohol and drug use, and sexual behaviours in street children of greater Cairo and Alexandra, Egypt. *Journal of AIDS, 24*(Suppl 2), 39–44. doi:10.1097/01.aids.0000386732.02425.d1.

Natural Resources and Agriculture Team of the United Kingdom, & Farrington, J. (2004). *Recognising and addressing risk and vulnerability constraints to pro-poor agricultural growth* (Report with Overseas Development Institute). Retrieved from http://dfid-agriculture-consultation.nri.org/summaries/wp6.pdf

Ndirangu, J., Bärnighausen, T., Tanser, F., Tint, K., & Newell, M. L. (2009). Levels of childhood vaccination coverage and the impact of maternal HIV status on child vaccination status in rural Kwazulu-Natal, South Africa. *Journal of Tropical Medicine and International Health, 14*(11), 1383–1393. doi:10.1111/j.1365-3156.2009.02382.x.

Nelson Mandela Foundation & Human Science Research Council. (2002). *South Africa prevalence, behavioural risks and mass media.* Cape Town: Human Science Research Council.

Neubauer, D., & Barbara, S. (2005). *Globalization, rapid urbanization and health infrastructure.* Santa Barbara: UCLA Global Research Center.

Newman, I., & Benz, C. R. (1998). *Qualitative-quantitative research methodology: Exploring the interactive continuum.* Carbondale: Southern Illinois University Press.

Nonnemaker, J. M., McNeely, C., A., & Blum, R. W. (2003). Public and private domains of religiosity and adolescent health risk behaviors: Evidence from the National Longitudinal Study of Adolescent Health. *Social Science and Medicine, 57*(11), 2049–2054.

Norman, F. (1991). The social construction of noncompliance: A study health care and social service providers in everyday practice. *Sociology of Health & Illness, 13*(3), 344–373. doi:10.1111/1467-9566.ep10492252.

Nutting, J. B. (2011). *Different stages in an addiction cycle.* Retrieved from http://www.voice-dialogue-inner-self-awareness.com/addictions16.html

Obeng, G. S., Kodzi, I., Emina, J., Adjei, J., & Ezeh, A. (2014). Adolescents sexual risk-taking in the informal settlements of Nairobi, Kenya: Understanding the contribution of religion. *Journal of Religion and Health, 53*(1), 13–26. doi:10.1007/s10943-012-9580-2.

Oldewage-Theron, W. H., Dicks, E. G., & Napier, C. E. (2006). Poverty household food insecurity and nutrition: Coping strategies in an informal settlement in the Vaal Triangle, South Africa. *Public Health, 120*(9), 795–804. doi:10.1016/j.puhe.2006.02.009.

Omololu, F. O., & Odutolu, O. (2007). HIV risk perception and constraints to protective behaviour among young slum dwellers. *Journal of Health Population Nutrition, 25*(2), 146–57. Retrieved from http://www.ncbi.nlm.nih.gov/pubmed/17985816

Onwugbuzie, A. J., & Leech, N. L. (2006). Linking research questions to mixed methods data analysis and procedure. *The Qualitative Report, 11*(3), 474–498. Retrieved from http://www.nova.edu/ssss/QR/QR11-3/onwuegbuzie.pdf

Oronje, R., Ndakala, J. C., Theobald, S., Lithur, N. A., & Ibisomi, L. (2011). Operationalizing sexual and reproductive health and rights in sub-Saharan Africa: Constraints, dilemma's and strategies. *BioMed Centre, International Health and Human Rights, 11,* 8. doi:10.1186/1472-698X-11-S3-S8.

Oti, A. O., & Kyobutungi, C. (2010). Verbal autopsy interpretation: A comparative analysis of the interval model versus physician review in determining causes of death in the Nairobi DSS. *Population Health Metrics, 8*(21). doi:10.1186/1478-7954-8-21.

Oti, S., Van de Vijver, S., & Aboderin, I. (2015). *Hypertension could be the new epidemic in Africa.* Retrieved from http://aphrc.org/hypertension-could-be-the-new-epidemic-in-africa/

Otoide, V. O., Orosanye, F., & Okonofua, F. (2001). Why Nigeria adolescents seek abortion rather than contraception: Evidence from focus-group discussion. *International Family Planning Perspectives, 27*(2). doi:10.2307/2673818.

Parker, R. G. (2000). Structural barriers and facilitators in HIV preventive: A review of international research. *AIDS, 14*(Suppl 1), 22–32. Retrieved from http://www.sfsu.edu/~multsowk/title/453.htm

Partners in Population Development (PPD). (2012). *Evidence for action: South-south collaboration for ICPD beyond 2014.* Paper presented at the PPD conference. Ruposhi Bangla Hotel, Dhaka. Abstract retrieved from http://pdfozz.net/k-33310811.html

Philipson, T. J., & Jena, A. B. (2006). Who benefits from New Medical Technologies? Estimates of consumer and producer surpluses for HIV/AIDS drugs. *Forum for Health Economics & Policy, 9*(2), 1558–9544. doi:10.2202/1558-9544.1005.

Pierre-Richard, A., & Canuto, A. (2013). *Gender equality and economic growth in Brazil. Poverty reduction and economic management(prem) network.* Retrieved from www.worldbank.org/economicpremise

Poudel, K. C., Jimba, M., Okumura, J., Anand, B. J., & Wakai, S. (2004). Migrants' risky sexual behaviours in India and at home in far western Nepal. *Tropical Medicine and International Health, 9*(8), 897–903. Retrieved from http://www.ncbi.nlm.nih.gov/pubmed/15303995

Quigley, M. A., Chandramohan, D., & Rodrigues L. C. (1999). Diagnostic accuracy of physician review, expert algorithms and data derived algorithms in adult verbal autopsies. *Journal of Epidemiology, 28,* 1081–1087. Retrieved from http://www.ncbi.nlm.nih.gov/pubmed/10661651

Refugee Consortium of Kenya. (2008). *Enhancing the protection the refugee women in Nairobi, a survey on risks protection gaps and coping mechanism of refugee women in urban areas.* Retrieved from the website of the Refugee Consortium of Kenya: http://www.rckkenya.org/rokdownloads/research/Enhancing%20Protection%20of%20Refugee%20Women.pdf

Report of the Australian Government Department of Families, Housing, Community Services and Indigenous Affairs. Retrieved from https://www.dss.gov.au/housing-Support

Richard, A. C., Cooper, A. M., McGinley, E. L., Fan, X., & Rosenthal, J. T. (2012). Poverty, wealth and health care utilization: A geographic assessment. *Urban Health: Bulletin of the New York Academy of Medicine, 89*(5), 5. doi:10.1007/s11524-012-9689-3.

Richter, L. M., Sherr, L., Adato, M., Belsey, M., Chandan, U., Desmond, C., Drimie, S., Haour-Knipe, M., Hosegood, V., Kimou, J., Madhavan, S., Mathambo, V., & Wakhweya, A. (2009). Strengthening families to support children affected by HIV/AIDS. *AIDS Care, 1*(Suppl 21), 3–12. doi:10.1080/09540120902923121.

Robert, J. K., Gray, R. H., Sewankambo, N. K., Serwadda, D., Wabwire-Mangen, F., Lutalo, T., & Wawer, J. M. (2003). Age differences in sexual partners and risk of HIV-1 infection in rural Uganda. *Journal of Acquired Immune Deficiency Syndromes, 32,* 446–451. Retrieved from http://www.ncbi.nlm.nih.gov/pubmed/12640205

Roelen, K., & Shelmerdine, H. (2014). *Researching the linkages between social protection and children's care in Rwanda* (Technical Report). doi:10.13140/2.1.1741.1364.

Rogow, D., & Haberland, N. (2005). Sexuality and relationships education: Towards, social studies approach. *Sex Education, 5,* 333–334. Retrieved from http://eric.ed.gov/?id=EJ834474

Roseanne, N. N. (2014). Political battles on women's bodies: Post-election conflicts and violence against women in internally displaced persons camps in Kenya. *Societies without Borders, 9*(1), 48–68.

Rutter, M. (1993). Resilience: Some conceptual considerations. *Journal of Adolescents Health, 14,* 626–631. Retrieved from http://www.ncbi.nlm.nih.gov/pubmed/8130234

Ryan, S., Franzetta, K., & Manlove, J. (2007). Knowledge, perceptions, and motivations for contraception: Influence on teens' contraceptive consistency. *Youth Society.* doi:10.1177/0044118X06296907.

Sabrina, N. P. (2015). Child care in crisis. *Parents.* Retrieved from http://www.worldpolicy.org/child-care-crisis

Sakar, N. N. (2008). Barriers to condom use. *The European Journal of Contraception & Reproductive Health Care, 13*(2), 114–122. doi:10.1080/13625180802011302.

Salo, E. (2005, January 26–27). *Ganging practices in Manenberg, South Africa and the ideologies of masculinity, gender and generational relations.* Paper presented at the conference "From boys to men: Masculinities & risk," University of the Western Cape. Abstract retrieved from http://www.csvr.org.za/wits/confpaps/salo.htm

Sampson, R. J., Morenoff, J. D., & Earls, F. (1999). Intelligence quotient scores of 4 year old children: Socialenvironmentalriskfactors.*Paediatrics,79*,343–350.doi:10.1046/j.1533-2500.2001.01011-79.x.

Santelli, J. S., Anderson, J. E., & Lindberg, L. D. (2006). Contraceptive use and pregnancy risk among U.S. high school students, 1991–2003. *Perspectives on Sexual and Reproductive Health, 38*(2), 106–111. Retrieved from http://www.guttmacher.org/pubs/journals/3810606.html

Sara, P., Elhawary, S., & Pantuliano, S. (2010, March). *Hidden and exposed: Urban refugees in Nairobi, Kenya* (HPG Working Paper). Retrieved from HPG website: http://www.odi.org/sites/odi.org.uk/files/odi-assets/publications-opinion-files/5858.pdf

Schmidt, B., & Schroder, I. (2001). *Anthropology of violence and conflict.* London: Routledge.

Scott-Sheldon, L. A., Huedo-Medina, T. B., Warren, M. R., Johnson, B. T., & Carey, M. P. (2011). Efficacy of behaviour interventions to increase condom use and reduce sexually transmitted infections. *Journal of Acquired Immune Deficiency Syndrome, 15, 58*(5), 489–498. doi:10.1097/QAI.0b013e31823554d7.

Setel, P. W., Whiting, D. R., Hemed, Y., Chandramohan, D., Wolfson, L. J., Alberti, K. G. M. M., & Lopez, A. D. (2006). Validity of verbal autopsy procedures for determining cause of death in Tanzania. *Tropical Medical and International Health, 11*(5), 681–696.

Setel, P. W., Macfarlane, S. B., Szreter, S., Mikkelsen, L., Jha, P., Stout, S., & Abouzahr, C. (2007). A scandal of invisibility, making everyone count by counting everyone. *The Lancet, 370*(9598), 1569–1577. doi:10.1016/S0140-6736(07)61307-5.

Sheehan, K. L. E., & Galvin, J. P., Jr. (2004). Urban children's perceptions of violence. *Archives of Pediatrics Adolescents Medicine, 158*(1), 74–77. doi:10.1001/archpedi.158.1.74.

Sheehan, K., Diacara, J. A., LeBailly, S., & Christoffel, K. K. (1997). Children's exposure to violence in urban setting. *Archives of Pediatric Adolescent Medicine, 151*(5), 502–504.

Sherr, L., Croome, N., Bradshaw, K., & Castaneda, K. P. (2014). A systematic review examining whether interventions are effective in reducing cognitive delay in children infected and affected with HIV/AIDS (Special Issue). *AIDS Care: Psychological and Socio-medical Aspects of AIDS/HIV, 26*(1). doi:10.1080/09540121.2014.906560.

Shrivastava, P. S., & Shrivasta, S. R. (2013). A study of spousal domestic violence in an urban slum of Mumbai. *International Journal of Preventive Medicine, 4*(1), 27–32. Retrieved from http://www.ncbi.nlm.nih.gov/pmc/articles/PMC3570908/

Singh, S., Darroch, J. E., & Bankole, A. (2003). *A, B and C in Uganda: The roles of abstinence, monogamy and condom use in HIV decline* (Occasional Report No 9). New York: The Alan Gettmacher Institute.

Sjostrand, M., Quist, V., Jacobson, A., Bergstrom, S., & Rogo, K. O. (1995). Socio-economic client characteristics and consequences of abortion in Nairobi. *East Africa Medical Journal, 72*(5), 325–332. Retrieved from https://www.researchgate.net/publication/15643008_Socio-economic_client_characteristics_and_consequences_of_abortion_in_Nairobi

Skinner, D., Tsheko, N., Mtero-Munyati, S., Segwabe, M., Chibatamoto, P., Mfecane, S., Chandiwana, B., Nkomo, N., Tlou, S., & Chitiyo, G. (2006). Towards a definition of orphaned and vulnerable children. *AIDS and Behavior, 10*(6), 619–626. Retrieved from http://www.ncbi.nlm.nih.gov/pubmed/16639543

Smith, D. J. (2000). These girls today and war: Premarital sexuality and modern identity in southeastern Nigeria. *Africa Today, Sexuality and Generational Identities in Sub-Saharan Africa, 47*(3/4), 99–120. Retrieved from http://www.jstor.org/stable/4187370

Smith, D. J. (2004). Youth, sin, sex in Nigeria: Christianity and HIV/AIDS-related beliefs and behavior among rural–urban migrants. *Culture, Health and Sexuality, 6*(5), 425–437. Retrieved from http://www.jstor.org/stable/4005308

Sommers, M. (2001). *Peace education and refugee youth.* Washington, DC: Jesuit Refugee Services.

Speizer, I. S., Fotso, J. C., Davis, J. T., Saad, A., & Otai, J. (2013). Timing and circumstances of first sex among female and male youth from selected urban areas of Nigeria, Kenya and Senegal. *Journal of Adolescent Health, 53*(5), 609–616. doi:10.1016/j.jadohealth.2013.06.004.

Spiegel, P. B., Bennedsen, A. R., Class, J., Bruns, L., Patterson, N., Yiweza, D., & Schilperoord, M. (2007). Prevalence of HIV infection in conflict-affected and displaced people in seven sub-Saharan African countries: A systematic review. *Lancet, 369*(9580), 2187–2195. Retrieved from http://www.ncbi.nlm.nih.gov/pubmed/17604801

Statman, D. (2000). Humiliation, dignity and self-respect. *Philosophical Psychology, 13*(4), 523–540. doi:10.1080/09515080020007643.

Steven, B. K., Williams, G. M., Najman, J. M., & Alati, R. (2013). Exploring the female specific risk to partial and full PTSD following physical assault. *Journal of Trauma Stress, 26*(1), 86–93. doi:10.1002/jts.21776.

Tarantola, D. (Ed.). (2000). Reducing HIV/AIDS risk, impact and vulnerability. *Bulletin WHO. 78*(2), 236–237. Retrieved from http://www.ncbi.nlm.nih.gov/pmc/articles/PMC2560688/ WHO

The Coalition of Children Affected by AIDS. (2014). *The Melbourne statement on young children born into HIV-affected famillies.* Retrieved from http://www.ccaba.org/the-melbourne-statement/

The Free Dictionary. (n.d.). Retrieved from http://www.thefreedictionary.com/addiction

The Global Fund. (2005). *Annual report, 2005. The global fund.* Retrieved from: http://www.the-globalfund.org/En/about/publications/annualreport2005/

The Global Fund. (2012). *The global fund to fight AIDS, tuberculosis and malaria.* Retrieved from http://www.one.org/us/policy/the-global-fund-to-fight-aids-tb-and-malaria/

Thea, D. W., Patel, L., Korth, M., & Forrester, C. (2008). *Johannesburg poverty and livelihood study.* Retrieved from http://www.ncr.org.za/pdfs/research reports/livelihoods%20study.pdf

Todd, E. (1996). Health inequalities in urban areas: A guide to the literature. *Journal of Environment and Urbanization, 8,* 141–152.

Tomas, J. P., & Jena, B. A. (2006). *Who benefits from new medical technologies? Estimates of consumer and producer surpluses for HIV/AIDS drugs* (Working Papers Series No. 11810). doi:10.3386/w11810.

Tord, K., Friel, S., Dixon, J., Corvalan, C., Rehfuess, E., Campbell-Lendrum, D., Gore, F., & Bartrum, J. (2007). Urban environmental health hazards and health equity. *Journal of Urban Health,* (Suppl 1), 8486–8497. Retrieved from http://www.ncbi.nlm.nih.gov/pubmed/17450427

Tually, S., Faulkner, D., & Thwaites-Tregilgas, E. (2012). *Instability in the housing circumstances of newly arrived humanitarian entrants and the implications for the homelessness service system: A scoping study* (Evidence Note No. 32). Retrieved from https://www.dss.gov.au/housing-support

United Nations. (2006). *The millenium development goals report 2006.* Retrieved from http://mdgs.un.org/unsd/mdg/Resources/Static/Products/Progress2006/MDGReport2006.pdf

United Nations. (2012). *The future we want. Rio + outcome document.* Retrieved from http://www.uncsd2012.org/thefuturewewant.html

United Nations. (2013a). *The millenium development goals report 2013.* Retrieved from http://www.un.org/millenniumgoals/pdf/report-2013/mdg-report-2013-english.pdf

United Nations. (2013b). *A new global partnership: Eradicate poverty and transform economies through sustainable development. The report of the high-level panel of eminent persons on the post-2015 development agenda.* Retrieved from http://www.un.org/sg/management/pdf/HLP_P2015_Report.pdf

United Nations Children's Fund (UNICEF). (2004). *Direct cash subsidy to orphans and other children made vulnerable by HIV/AIDS. Pilot project.* Retrieved from http://www.unicef.org/publications/index_51775.html

United Nations Children's Fund (UNICEF). (2009). *State of the world's children (special edition) statistical tables.* Retrieved from http://www.unicef.org/publications/index_51775.html

United Nations Children's Fund (UNICEF). (2011). *UNICEF annual report 2011.* New York: UNICEF.

United Nations Children's Fund (UNICEF) & Children Welfare Society of Kenya. (2008). *Separated children in Kenya.* Unpublished manuscript.

United Nations Children's Fund (UNICEF), Joint United Nations Programme on HIV/AIDS (UNAIDS), World Health Organization (WHO) & United Nations Fund Population Fund (UNFPA). (2010). *Children and AIDS: Fifth stocktaking report*. Retrieved from http://www.unicef.org/publications/files/Children_and_AIDS-Fifth_Stocktaking_Report_2010_EN.pdf

United Nations Children's Fund (UNICEF), President's Emergency Plan for AIDS Relief (PEPFAR), Joint United Nations Programme on HIV/AIDS (UNAIDS), United States Agency for International Development (USAID), The World Bank & The Coalition for Children Affected by AIDS. (2014, July 20). *Protection, care and support for an AIDS-free generation: A call to action for all children*. Retrieved from http://www.childrenandaids.org/css/GPF-2014-Call-to-Action(1).pdf

United Nations Department of Economics and Social Affairs. (2009). *World population prospects: The 2009 revision population database*. Retrieved from http://esa.un.org/unpd/wup/

United Nations Department of Economic and Social Affairs. (2014). *World urbanization prospects: 2014 revision: Highlights*. Retrieved from http://esa.un.org/undp/wup/

United Nations Fund Population Fund (UNFPA). (2015). *The inter agency task team (IATT) on HIV and young people in humanitarian emergencies. Brief*. Retrieved from www.unfpa.org/hiv/iattdocs/humanitarian.pdf

United Nations General Assembly. (2013). *Outcome document of the special event towards achievening the millennium development goals*. Retrieved from http://www.un.org/en/ga/search/view doc.asp?symbol=A/68/L.4

United Nations High Commissioner for Human Rights. (2008, February 6–28). *Report from United Nations High Commissioner for Human Rights, fact-finding mission to Kenya*. Retrieved from http://www.ohchr.org/Documents/Press/OHCHRKenyareport.pdf

United Nations High Commissioner for Refugees (UNHCR). (2007). *Refugee and Asylum seekers in Kenya. Internally displaced persons: Questions and answers*. Retrieved from http://www.unhcr.org/cgi-bin/texis/vtx/home

United Nations High Commissioner for Refugees (UNHCR). (2009). *UNHCR policy on refugee protection and solutions in urban areas*. Retrieved from http://www.refworld.org/docid/4ab8e7f72.html

United Nations High Commissioner for Refugees (UNHCR) & World Health Organization (WHO). (2008). *The right to health* (Fact Sheet No. 31). Retrieved from http://www.ohchr.org/EN/PublicationsResources/Pages/FactSheets.aspx

United Nations Human Settlements Programme (UN–Habitat). (2004). *The state of the world's cities 2004/5. Globalization and urban culture*. Retrieved from http://www.amazon.co.uk/State-Worlds-Cities-2004-Globalization/dp/184407160X

United Nations Office for Disaster Risk Reduction – Regional Office for Africa (UNISDR). (2014, May 13–16). *Declaration of the fifth African regional platform for disaster risk reduction*. Abuja. Retrieved from http://www.preventionweb.net/english/hyogo/regional/platform/afrp/2014/

United Nations Population Information Network (POPIN), United Nations Population Division, Department of Economic and Social Affairs & United Nations Population Fund (UNFPA). (1994). *Guidelines on reproductive health*. Retrieved from http://www.un.org/popin/unfpa/taskforce/guide/iatfreph.gdl.html

United States Agency for International Development (USAID). (2004). *Improving the health of the urban poor: Learning from USAID experience* (Strategic Report No. 12). Washington, DC: USAID.

Vold, G., & Bernard, T. (1986). *Theoretical criminology*. New York: Oxford University Press.

Wadhwa, V. (2012). Structural violence and women's vulnerability to HIV/AIDS in India: Understanding through a "grief model" framework. *Annals of the Association of American Geographers, 102*(5), 1200–1208. doi:10.1080/00045608.2012.659966.

Wanyeki, M. (2008). Lessons from Kenya: Women and the post-elections violence. *Feminist Africa: Militarism, Conflict and Women's Activism*. Retrieved from http://www.iiav.nl/ezines/web/FeministAfrica/2008

Watkins, R. (2008). *Fighting climate change: Human security in a divided world*. Retrieved from https://www.google.com/search?q=Fighting+Climate+change%3A+Human+security+in+a+Divided+world&oq=Fighting+Climate+change%3A+Human+security+in+a+Divided+world&aqs=chrome..69i57.14263j0j4&sourceid=chrome&es_sm=93&ie=UTF-8

Weiss, R. (2001). Gulliver's travel in HIV land. *Nature, 410*, 963–967. doi:10.1038/35073632.

Weiss, R. A., & McLean, A. R. (2003). What have we learnt from SARS? *Philosophical Transcripts of the Royal Society London B: Biological Sciences, 359*, 1137–1140.

Welti, K., Wildsmith, E., & Manlove, J. (2006). Trends and recent estimates: Contraceptive use among U.S. teens. *Child Trends, 2011*(23). Retrieved from http://www.childtrends.org/?publications=trends-and-recent-estimates-contraceptive-use-among-u-s-teens-and-young-adults

Wordsworth, M. (2015, April 20). HIV: Rapid testing, preventative drugs used in the fight against Queensland's rising infection rate. *ABC News*. Retrieved from http://www.abc.net.au/news/2015-03-16/ experts-attacking-queenslands-rising-hiv-infection-rate/6323880

World Food Programme (WFP), United States Agency for International Development (USAID) & CARE. (2008). *Field methods manual*. Retrieved from http://wfpusa.org/

World Health Organisation (WHO). (1999). *Programming for adolescent health and development*. Retrieved from http://www.who.int/maternal_child_adolescent/documents/trs_886/en/

World Health Organisation (WHO). (2003a). *Community contribution to TB care: Practice and policy*. Retrieved from https://www.google.com/url?sa=t&rct=j&q=&esrc=s&source=web&cd =1&cad=rja&uact=8&ved=0CB0QFjAA&url=http%3A%2F%2Fwhqlibdoc.who. int%2Fhq%2F2003%2FWHO_CDS_TB_2003.312.pdf&ei=M18zVfffK8HTaKvegfAP&usg =AFQjCNHA_vIhgZ8ZHwnUNlUWwR_LbHWyyw&bvm=bv.91071109,d.d2s

World Health Organisation (WHO). (2003b). *The world health report 2003*. Retrieved from http://www.who.int/whr/2003/en/

World Health Organisation (WHO). (2005a). *Towards a conceptual framework for analysis and action on the social determinants of health: Discussion paper for the commission on the social determinants of health*. Retrieved from http://www.naccho.org/topics/justice/resources/upload/WHOCommissionTowardsConceptualFrame.pdf

World Health Organisation (WHO). (2005b). *Addressing poverty in TB control: Options for national TB control programmes*. Retrieved from http://www.who.int/tb/challenges/poverty/en/

World Health Organisation (WHO). (2007). *The health of the African people. The African regional health report*. Retrieved from http://www.who.int/bulletin/africanhealth/en/index.html

World Health Organisation (WHO). (2008a). *Our cities our health our future: Acting on social determinants for health equity in urban settings*. Retrieved from http://www.who.int/social_determinants/resources/knus_report_16jul07.pdf

World Health Organisation (WHO). (2008b). *Primary health care now more than ever*. Retrieved from http://www.who.int/whr/2008/en/

World Health Organisation (WHO), Joint United Nations Programme on HIV/AIDS (UNAIDS) & United Nations Children's Fund (UNICEF). (2007). *Towards universal access, scaling up priority HIV/AIDS interventions in the health sector*. Retrieved from http://www.who.int/hiv/pub/2010progressreport/en/

World Health Organisation (WHO), Joint United Nations Programme on HIV/AIDS (UNAIDS) & United Nations Children's Fund (UNICEF). (2009). *Epidemiological fact sheet of HIV and AIDS/Kenya*. Retrieved from http://data.unaids.org/Publications/Fact-Sheets01/Kenya_EN.pdf

Zaryab, I., & Christopher, Z. (2011). Violent conflict and the spread of HIV/AIDS in Africa. *The Journal of Politics, 72*(1), 149–162. doi:10.1017/S0022381609990533.

Zheng, Z. L. (2005, July 18–33). *Health vulnerability among temporary migrants in urban China*. Paper presented at the XXV international population conference. Abstract retrieved from http://iussp2005.princeton.edu/papers/51980

Ziraba, A. K., Madise, N. J., Matilu, M., Zulu, E., Kebaso, J., Khamidi, S., Okoth, V. & Ezeh, C. (2010). The effect of participant nonresponse on HIV prevalence estimates in a population-based survey in two informal settlements in Nairobi city. *Population Health Metrics, 8*, 22. Retrieved from http://www.pophealthmetrics.com/content/8/1/22

Zlidar, V., Gardner, R., Rutstein, S. O., Morris, L. & Goldberg, H. (2003). *New survey findings: The reproductive revolution continues*. Retrieved from http://www.popline.org/node/193091#sthash.K1D0iPzL.dpuf

Printed in the United States
By Bookmasters